THE HIGHEST HURDLE

THE HIGHEST HURDLE

An ALS Journey of Faith, Laughter, Love and Friendship

Kim Wroblewski

ELM HILL

A Division of
HarperCollins Christian Publishing

www.elmhillbooks.com

© 2019 Kim Wroblewski

The Highest Hurdle
An ALS Journey of Faith, Laughter, Love and Friendship

All rights reserved. No portion of this book may be reproduced, stored in a retrieval system, or transmitted in any form or by any means—electronic, mechanical, photocopy, recording, scanning, or other—except for brief quotations in critical reviews or articles, without the prior written permission of the publisher.

Published in Nashville, Tennessee, by Elm Hill, an imprint of Thomas Nelson. Elm Hill and Thomas Nelson are registered trademarks of HarperCollins Christian Publishing, Inc.

Elm Hill titles may be purchased in bulk for educational, business, fund-raising, or sales promotional use. For information, please e-mail SpecialMarkets@ ThomasNelson.com.

Library of Congress Cataloging-in-Publication Data

Library Congress Control Number: 2018965716

ISBN 978-0-310101833 (Paperback)
ISBN 978-0-310101840 (Hardbound)
ISBN 978-0-310101857 (eBook)

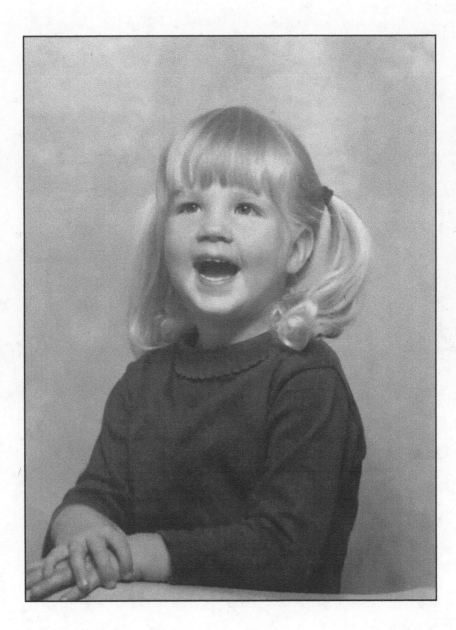

INTRODUCTION

If you bought this book, we sincerely thank you! We hope you laugh, cry, and discover a deeper faith. Most importantly, we hope you discover that life is short and that if you are dealt a crappy hand, it does not mean you have to throw in the towel and give up. You can live a positive and happy life and make a lasting impact on others. We are not "come to Jesus, in your face Christians." We are both, we think, funny, optimistic, hardworking, fantastic moms (our children will totally agree with this), and we live for our families. Our goal is to help people find treatments, diets, and to show how our wonderful support group functioned, while remaining positive in a horrible situation—as well as sharing and growing through our faith, in which we have been incredibly blessed. We hope you enjoy the journey. All proceeds are going to pay for ALS medical treatments for people in the Northern Michigan area, and hopefully scholarships for some well-deserving kids!

Thank you and God bless!
MaryFran Kolp and Kim Wroblewski

PART 1

MEETING MARYFRAN

MaryFran and I laughed about how we met in 1997. She was working at the local hospital, doing health screenings. I decided to go one day and have my fat calipered, as I have always struggled with my weight and prefer to be referred to as "curvy." MaryFran—a six-foot tall, blond, beautiful, athletic, smiling, and energetic woman—happily obliged to pinch my fat. Being very outgoing people (meaning we talk a lot), we started talking and found that not only did we have a lot in common, we lived within two miles of each other out in the country. Little did we know that this meeting would result in a long-lasting friendship, better known as *sisterhood*. Through the years, we would watch each other's children, carpool, and volunteer together for different organizations. We also attended the same church, sent our kids to the same schools, and had very similar parenting styles. Our husbands worked together at the same hospital and also had similar interests.

The most amazing thing about MaryFran was that she was the most positive person anyone would ever meet. You instantly become her friend. It didn't matter what the situation was; she would find the silver lining. If something bad happened in your life, she would be the first one at your door with a meal, or a card would show up in your mailbox. She even took in my dog with two broken legs for a weekend so that we wouldn't lose out on tickets we had for a University of Michigan football game. The crazy thing was when we came home, he didn't want to leave her side! She had this amazing sense of humor, too. After I had my hysterectomy and had issues with my bladder, she of course was the first one to come over with food and noticed the urine in my catheter bag was quite an unusual color. She did not know I was on medication that changed the color of my urine. She said to me when she was leaving, "Hey, not sure if you noticed, but your urine is a really funky color and you might want to get that checked out!" Before texting, we would spend hours on the phone, sharing wisdom or talking about our children, school, etc. We tag-teamed for our church funeral lunches, which of course she told me about and talked me into doing. We were co-presidents of the Northern Michigan Medical Society Alliance and active members for years. We spent many hours together volunteering for St. Francis Xavier School and Church, and she was one of my most cherished friends. She was one of my few friends who, if I called in an emergency, she would drop whatever she was doing and just be there for me.

NORTHERN MICHIGAN

Petoskey is a tiny resort community nestled on the shores of Little Traverse Bay in Northern Michigan. Michiganders use their hands as a map to show where they are from; Petoskey would be at the edge of the top of your ring finger! Locals joke that you can find many unique and beautiful gifts but not a pair of underwear in our town!

Summers in Petoskey are known for "million-dollar" sunsets, Petoskey stones (our state stone), fudge, ice cream, art, gorgeous sandy beaches, festivals, and our Fourth of July Parade, where practically the whole town turns out and stays for our spectacular fireworks display over the bay. It is common to see people at our beachfront park biking, walking, playing softball, checking out the boats in the marina, or just napping in the grass. The kids and some brave adults will be jumping off the Petoskey lighthouse break-wall into the ice-cold, sparkling, blue Lake Michigan water to cool off on warm days. You will always see people's backsides in the air in the familiar "Petoskey stone stoop" along the shoreline, searching for the elusive Petoskey stone for a keepsake to take home. If you are lucky, a local may take pity on you and show you how it's done. (You should look in the water, as it's easier to see the coral pattern when the stones are wet. You are welcome.) The Petoskey waterfront is so beautiful that it is often painted by local artists with St. Francis Xavier Church as a focal point. The church has been a major landmark since the late 1800s. Our town's population easily triples in the summer with the snowbirds and with our many summer tourists (snowbirds are Michiganders that leave the harsh winters for warmer climates like Florida or Arizona and come back in the late spring). Petoskey is also lucky to have many family farms, some of them organic, that bring their wares in town on Fridays to sell at our farmer's market.

Fall brings spectacular colors of gold, maroon, and orange, and people come on foliage tours to see our beautiful area. The whole town turns out to watch football on Friday nights and everyone knows everyone. Our school is very fortunate to have a brand-new stadium that rivals some of the best downstate elite schools after years of hosting games in a run-down stadium that we still packed to the rafters. We cheer on the sports teams winning or losing. The marching band has been winning awards for over thirty years and the joke is when the football team has a losing season, everyone is there to watch the band at half-time. Even the opposing team's fans come over to watch our band. Our sports teams have had many successful seasons. Petoskey High School families travel for their teams and we travel far. Our teams play in towns as far away as Escanaba (in the upper peninsula), a four-hour drive; Grand Rapids, a three-hour drive; Alpena, a two-hour drive; and Traverse City, just over an hour's drive. For people who don't live in Michigan, we tell how far away something is by how long it takes to drive it, not by how many miles. If your kid is on a sports team, you can be sure that if they played well, you will definitely hear about it. It is very common for them to appear in the sport section of the local paper and people will cut them out and save them for you. November 15 is considered a holiday, as it is opening day for deer-hunting season. Men and a lot of women, many with their kids, head into the woods to get the big buck; a nice one in Northern Michigan is usually eight points or more. If you get a nice one, the men are always eager to tell how many points their buck had and show you a photo of their son or daughter with their first deer.

Winters are not for the weak of heart in Northern Michigan. They can start as early as Halloween and last till Mother's Day. The average winter produces over a hundred inches of snow a year and some have had seasons with over 200 inches of snow. We get the lovely "lake effect" snow, and when it comes it comes down hard and fast. If the sun comes out in the winter, everyone says wow, what a beautiful day today! Rarely is school canceled and Petoskey High School is almost always the last one to close. Skiing and snowboarding are essential to learn at an early age to cope with the long winter, and we are fortunate to have three ski resorts nearby. As I am writing this we are in the middle of a huge snow-storm and it is April 14!

Sometimes we get to experience the ever-elusive spring season. It is a really long winter, and then boom, it is summer. The saying goes "if you don't like the weather in Michigan, wait an hour and it will change." If it is 50 degrees in the spring, we will put on our shorts and be ready to go outdoors. May brings out the morel-mushroom hunters into the woods. Morels are a delicious mushroom native to our woods, and locals do not like to share their secret spots!

Northern Michigan people are hardy folks. It is a great place to live and raise kids. The people are friendly and helpful. Whenever I make the drive into town and I see the bay, its beauty never ceases to amaze me.

EARLY YEARS

MaryFran grew up in South Lyon, Michigan, a suburb of Detroit. Dan and Carole Peterlin gave her a wonderful childhood. They supported her and her sister Natalie in everything that they did. They were always active in their church. A devout Catholic, she received her sacraments and participated in youth group. In 1984, MaryFran was chosen to represent her church to attend one of the first World Youth Days. On this trip she saw Pope John II coming, within five feet of his car. Fran was also able to meet Mother Teresa and got to listen to her talk about her work with the poor. She attended the Stations of the Cross at the Colosseum church service at St. Paul's Basilica on a Friday night, and went to the tomb of St. Francis at Assisi. MaryFran also toured the ruins of Rome and the Sistine Chapel. It was an amazing experience for a young Catholic lady and made a lasting impact on her life.

She was very athletic. To say sports played a huge part in her life is an understatement. As early as middle school she excelled in sports and was raking in the trophies and ribbons. She once told me that if they were allowed to watch television, when commercials were on her dad made them do sit-ups and push-ups. No sitting around for the Peterlin girls! Recently, she was inducted into the South Lyon High School Athletic Hall of Fame. She played on the varsity basketball team for three years, competed on the varsity volleyball team for three years, and participated on the varsity track and field for four years. The records she set at her high school for the 4 × 400-meter relay, 330-meter hurdles, and 100-meter hurdles remain to this day.

Grand Valley State University in Grand Rapids, Michigan, offered her an academic scholarship, and when she went there she was able to compete athletically. She competed in basketball for two years and track and field for four years. She went on to set eight records at GVSU. The records in the 50- and 100-meter hurdles are still standing. In 1990, she graduated with a dual major: Bachelor of Science in physical education and biology. She went on to earn a Master of Science and a PhD in exercise physiology with an emphasis in pediatrics from the University of Toledo.

MaryFran Peterlin met her future husband, Andy Kolp, by chance at a basketball practice. She was a freshman at Grand Valley State University and walked into the men's team practice with her mentor before her own practice. She saw Andy, turned to her mentor, and said, "I am going to marry those legs." Unbeknownst to her, her mentor was his girlfriend at the time! Fast forward ten years, they met again with a group of friends at Mr. Sports Bar in Bloomfield, Michigan. They started dating and fell in love. They married on August 16, 1996 at St. Patrick Catholic Church in Brighton, Michigan. In their wedding program was a special thank you:

Close families and good friendships are things to be cherished.
We thank you for joining in our special moment. God bless you.

Love,
MaryFran and Andy

They practiced this sentiment their whole married life.

That summer they moved to Northern Michigan, where Andy could start his career as an Emergency Room Physician. She started working as a wellness consultant at the Northern Michigan Hospital Foundation. MaryFran sought many grants with the hospital and diabetes staff for the development of cardiovascular disease risk interventions. She always had an interest in health and well-being. Their son Danny was born on June 14, 1999 and Megan followed on August 30, 2001. They were the ideal family.

The Kolps are a social family. They made many friends in a lot of different circles. They belong to St. Francis Xavier Church, they sent their children to St. Francis Xavier School and then on to Petoskey High School. Wherever they went, they actively volunteered and made new friends. Andy and MaryFran are known for inviting everyone to their house for get-togethers. MaryFran never liked to exclude anyone!

St. Francis Xavier School

St. Francis Xavier School is pretty much the meeting place for many of our friends. It is a fairly-small Catholic school, though you do not have to be Catholic to attend. They offer pre-k through eighth grade, averaging about 200 students. Every morning starts with daily prayer and one day a week is a school-wide mass. MaryFran and I loved going to the school mass. Father Denny mostly presided over these masses and he really did a great job talking directly to the kids. He has a wonderful sense of humor. I think a lot of his messages were aimed secretly at the parents who attended, too. My children and MaryFran's children have a very close relationship with this special priest, as do many of the kids at our school. Many of the parents attend this mass and a lot of our group of friends would go to breakfast afterward. It is very close-knit community.

At the school you were required to volunteer with playground duty, lunch duty, and help with the school's major fund-raiser. We all worked the gala auction, which was not only the major funding for our school but also the biggest event of the year, not just for our school but pretty much for Petoskey. It was always a great party with lots of dancing and revelry while celebrating our wonderful school. Most of us had chaired it and puts tons of hours making it work. Fran always liked to say we need your "time, talent, and treasure" to make it work, or "many hands make light work." She had a way of getting people "roped" into working. You could never say no to her. Occasionally, we would disagree but we would always work it out.

The great thing about the school, I think that most of the parents would say is that they have such a close relationship with the teachers after their children have gone there. I know my children and MaryFran's have gone back to visit the teachers, and so have their classmates. The teachers really care about the kids. We are very fortunate to have small class sizes and I think that really helps. MaryFran and I have always felt that you became friends with the teachers and staff.

St. Francis Xavier Church

The church was always a big part of MaryFran's life. St. Francis Xavier Church is the main Catholic church in Petoskey. It was founded in the late 1800s. Since 2001, Father Denny Stilwell has been leading our parish. He is a big supporter of our Catholic school and loves our children. He is very close with the Kolp family and with mine. He is funny and gives some great homilies. The Kolps have been very active members in the parish, from funeral lunches, Brother Dan's Pantry, lectors, greeters, ushers, faith formation, and youth group.

I honestly wish that my faith was as strong as hers. I try to work at my faith, but she always had this inner peace and devotion that I have rarely seen in anyone else. She was not the type of person who would preach at you and tell you that if you don't believe or if you're not Catholic you are going straight to hell. She would readily admit her faults. She had a great sense of humor about herself, but she was sneaky about how she evangelized. It might be a book she thought you might like or just a quote or maybe just hey, think about this. She always said we are a work in progress. Trust me, after you read this book, you will definitely have (I hope) a deeper sense of your own faith, or maybe you will think you need to work on your faith, just like I did.

CELEBRATIONS

MaryFran loved to celebrate! She would find any reason to have a party. Last day of school? Let's go to Petoskey State Park and have a picnic to celebrate that last day of school. September 11? Let's have a shot under the chandelier at her house and say a prayer for the people who lost their lives. Weddings? What a beautiful celebration of two people's love for each other. A new baby? That is the best reason to celebrate! A gift was on its way and she would be one of the first ones in line to hold that little bundle of joy. A child getting an award? She would be congratulating in some way; you could guarantee it. She would find any excuse to celebrate, no matter how small. She wasn't an "every child gets a participation ribbon" person but felt that if something was achieved it should be recognized.

BIRTHDAYS

S he started the after-kid drop-off at school, birthday-breakfast, and spa-day birthday celebrations. If it was your birthday, we were celebrating whether you wanted to or not. If you didn't want to celebrate, then you were surprised. Sorry, no choice in the matter. MaryFran was celebrating that you were born and that was that. There are a couple great little restaurants right by our little school that are prime gathering spots. Our favorites were The Bistro, which has since moved North of town and Julienne Tomatoes. Small gifts and funny cards were given and at The Bistro a silly birthday hat was sometime placed on your head. Of course, everyone had to sing! We enjoyed breakfast and everyone chipped in for the birthday girl. Spa days were another luxury. We would head off to Boyne Mountain for most of the day for a work-out, spa service and get lunch. It is a tradition that we of course continue in her honor to this day. We feel we must keep celebrating out of respect for MaryFran! It is a tough thing to keep doing but sacrifice we must!

You're Invited—You Can Say No, but You Won't...

One of the things MaryFran is famous for was her direct-sales parties. Over the years, she sold Discovery Toys, Arbonne, Madison Handbags, and Mona V. She mainly did this to get out of the house after she had kids. It was a way to get other women together who basically needed a much-needed break from their kids and husbands. While perusing the catalogs, we would have drinks and appetizers and just talk, a lot of girl talk. The nights would always have much-needed laugh and everyone would go home refreshed and feeling great! After a while, we started teasing her that she was always trying to sell us stuff. She just liked having people over.

HERSHEY BAR

As a coach, MaryFran was very inspirational. She did not believe in tearing down girls but building them up. Every year she coached, she gave the girls a Hershey bar. She told them that they each represented a piece of the bar. If a piece was missing from the bar, the team would not be complete. If the team was not complete, they would not be able to compete as a team, which meant that each girl was very important to the team.

ORGANIC COOKING CLUB

MaryFran was organic before organic became the "in" thing to do. I didn't really even know what organic was when I met her. I thought it was some hippy thing. I mean, it was the late 1990s. Who really cared then about eating pesticides? I just knew organic was expensive and hard to find in the grocery stores in Northern Michigan. Unless you went to this funky store where everyone had nose rings and dreadlocks. Sorry, not my scene, and it smelled weird in there with all the incense and stuff! The Grain Train has moved and it now looks like a normal grocery store—the kids still have nose rings and tattoos, but nowadays, who doesn't? I have joined now and go there frequently. See how she worked her Jedi mind tricks? Anyways, she had this idea about an organic cooking club and she talked Julie from Julienne Tomatoes into helping her get it started. They started in 2006 and it is still going to this day. They got together and cooked a bunch of meals to freeze for their families. It makes it easier for busy families to have healthy options ready to thaw, as the work is done in one night. The ladies decided to donate meals to the Kolp family as their way to give back.

LITTLE HOUSE, THE WALTONS, HALLMARK AND NCAA BASKETBALL

What do they all have in common? MaryFran loved to watch them. I used to tease her about watching them. She couldn't wait until Christmas, when the Hallmark channel would start airing all those sappy shows where you always knew they would have happy endings. I asked her one time how she could watch them when it was so easy to figure out what was going to happen, and the acting was mediocre. She said she just couldn't stand watching all those reality television shows with no values or morality. Fran said at least these shows showed good values and taught a good lesson at the end. She would always put out a text around Christmas, inviting friends over to watch the Hallmark channel Christmas shows.

Little House was probably her favorite show. I remember stopping over one time and she was crying. I asked her if anything was wrong and she said, sheepishly, that she almost always cried at the end of *Little House*. She loved that show. She loved that the families loved each other and that there was always a good moral to each episode.

I think the only other thing she loved to watch more was the Detroit Tigers and NCAA basketball. Look out during March madness. The Kolps were watching basketball and it didn't matter who was playing. They knew all the teams and all the players. They are huge Michigan State Spartan fans.

BAD NEWS

O ur circle of friends started to become concerned six months prior, when we noticed subtle changes. Sometimes MaryFran's speech would be a little slurred, which had several people asking if she had been drinking. One day she asked Deanna if she noticed if her speech sounded funny to her. She also noticed that sometimes she was having difficulties walking. Then there were the muscle twitches. She was a very strong-willed woman and was blowing off our concerns. Her husband Andy is an Emergency Room Physician as is his brother-in-law, and they were trying to get her to go get some testing done. She was in the middle of helping with our children's school auction and was just chalking it up to being tired and stressed. Finally, after the auction was over, several of her close friends got together and we knew we had to force the issue on her. I was designated the person to do the intervention as she seemed to listen to me better. I decided on sending a text because it would be "in her face" and she would have to read it. We had always been rather blunt with each other, more like sisters, so I knew if she got mad it would blow over quickly. I did not save the original text, but it went something like this:

Hi Fran, several of us are very concerned about your health. You can tell me go to hell, but I need to tell you this. I know if I were to talk to you, you would blow me off, so I am making you read this. I think you need to go to a neurologist and have some testing done. You need an EMG, muscle biopsy, and some basic neurological testing. I would not be telling you this if I didn't love you!

My friend Deanna and I, during a telephone conversation, decided to get online and do a differential diagnosis. We felt that based on her symptoms and our research she could have Lyme, multiple sclerosis, or ALS. Luckily, or not so lucky, my text worked, and she went and got tested.

July 3, 2014 will be a life-changing date forever. It was not just my girlfriend's forty-seventh birthday, but the day she received a devastating diagnosis of Amyotrophic Lateral Sclerosis (ALS). I will never forget receiving the text she sent and where I was. All her friends were patiently waiting, hoping it would be multiple sclerosis or Lyme disease. Both not great diagnoses but better than ALS. This was also the summer of the ALS ice-bucket challenge. A weird coincidence, to be sure. This began her ALS journey. Everyone who knows her will instantly recognize her "voice."

PART 2

PART 2

ALS JOURNEY

MaryFran decided she was not going to sit idly and let this disease ruin her life. She was known for grabbing the bull by the horns, jumping in, and tackling things. A friend told her about the CaringBridge app. This was a tool she could use for making journal entries and keeping friends and family up to date. Her first post was after her diagnosis. The first few entries were made by our friend Maggie Kromm. Maggie helped set up the app for MaryFran and would post for her until she had time to give her a tutorial on how to use the app.

Fourth of July Announcement

July 28, 2014
Posted by Maggie Kromm

MaryFran's announcement: Hello! Happy 4th and many blessings to all of you! Well here it is I have been surrounded by great friends and family this holiday season!!!! I in the midst was given some challenging news. I have ALS. I am going onto treatment and second opinions and Eastern and Western medicine. I am not in pain. Just a little shock and I talk funny! I ask for prayers which I know all of you will give me. Many of you are surrounded by loved ones, enjoy every moment! I have the best spouse EVER and best family and friends! I'll be talking with all of you soon but honestly couldn't decide who to call first. My kids know and are just starting to understand. Love y'all. xxoo

July 30, 2014
Journal entry by Maggie Kromm
(For MaryFran)

Hi Friends! I had my meeting with Dr. Perlmutter, a specialist in neurological disease disorders today and it appears the original diagnosis may be correct! Nevertheless, I have been put on all kinds of natural supplements, shots, injections … all natural of course and yes, I'm still walking!!! I have a bunch of reading to do and I'm excited to move forward with my life! Who would have thought that my doctorate would come in handy for my own personal case! Although, the outcome for this disease can look grim I always like to defy the odds! No, there is not a specific cause for ALS, therefore there are lot of areas that can contribute to this disease and I'm looking forward to tackling each of them one at a time! Don't be sad or surprised, after all this is what I do! The motto I live by is whatever it takes! And that's what I will do! Keep the prayers coming! I feel an inner sense of peace and I know many of you are praying for me and my family! I am here to do God's work! And this happens to be part of it! My kids are God's kids! I have been blessed with the best husband ever!! Awesome over the top friends and family… and what a blessed supportive community we live in! I have candles lit in churches burning for me that I've never visited! What else is there? For those given much, much will be asked! I'm up for the task! Now pull up your bootstraps and get on to business! It's a beautiful day and after all isn't one day at a time all we each get? Hugs to all of you!

I was at a loss. I mean, what do you do when your friend is given a death sentence? On my trip to Europe, I decided to light a candle in every church that I visited and say a prayer for MaryFran. This was not something I would normally do and was outside of my comfort zone, but I thought I was willing to do "whatever it takes" to help. I told myself that I was going to be strong for her and that I would not cry in front of her.

Treatment update

August 5, 2014

By Maggie Kromm - 3 years ago

MaryFran is down state having started hyperbaric treatments. She writes about the treatment: Good! Very interesting process so here I am at the hyperbaric center in South Lyon. As I get to be relaxed for an hour and 20 minutes while oxygen is infused into my system and finally get to watch Downtown Abbey!!! I'm through the first series! It's relaxing. I'll be doing treatments twice a day for 14 days! Interesting my symptoms are being more refined. All upper body, very minimal lower. Results between EMG at home and at U of M very different. Neurologist at U of M perplexed. U of M is doing a spinal and more blood tests on me next week. I'll keep u posted! Looks as if all my supplements are helping me? Hugs!

Hyperbaric treatments are when they put you in a special "cylinder" chamber for a certain amount of time and you receive increased amounts of oxygen. Some of the benefits are supposed to be:

Boosts supply of circulating stem cells, promote growth of new capillaries and blood vessels, boost efficacy of chemotherapy drugs, 77 percent increase in survival rates of patients with metastatic cancer when combined with the ketogenic diet, promote new nerve growth in the brain, reduce radiation-induced information and tissue and bones, stimulates oxygenation, and supports faster wound healing.

Letter from a young poet

August 7, 2014

By Maggie Kromm - 3 years ago

The following is one of MaryFran's favorites: *Be patient toward all that is unsolved in your heart and try to love the questions*

35

themselves. Do not now seek the answers, *which cannot be given you because you would not be able to live them. And the point is to live everything. Live the questions now. Perhaps you will then gradually, without noticing it, live along some distant day into the answers.* Rainer Maria Rilke

Bravelets
August18, 2014
By Maggie Kromm - 3 years ago

Please follow the link below to purchase a Bravelet item. $10 from each sale will go towards medical expenses for MaryFran. https://bravelets. com/bravepage/whatever-it-takes-for-maryfran-peterlin-kolp

MaryFran has always used the phrase "Whatever it Takes" in her support of our community. She has been active in coaching volleyball and basketball, raising funds for the St. Francis Xavier School and supporting Petoskey Athletics and our medical community. Recently, she has been given a health challenge and now it is our time to do "Whatever it Takes" to support her.

End of summer update
September 2, 2014
By Maggie Kromm - 3 years ago

From MaryFran:
Hello everyone! Here is a MaryFran update! First of all, I want to thank everyone for their participation or their thoughts and prayers and funds for the ALS ice bucket challenges! Businesses, families, kids and teens! They have been hilarious! And fun to watch despite the concerning situation! I can't believe over 95 million dollars have already been raised towards the research toward a cause and a cure! This past weekend we were part of a great

fundraising effort put on by the Northern Michigan Emergency Department it was a very touching event! As for what's going on for now with the Kolps were looking forward to a great start to a great school year! I will be heading downstate for additional hyperbaric treatments for the remainder of the week but will be back this coming weekend! In addition, most of my additional testing and follow-up appointments and results should be completed and we will officially be able to start moving forward! I'll keep all of you posted thank you for your continued thoughts and prayers!

Journal entry by Maggie Kromm — 9/15/2014

Hi friends of MaryFran. Please check out the PLANNER tab on this website to sign up for weekly dinners. These meals have no dietary restrictions and will be for Andy, Danny, Megan and the occasional parent or in-law. Please pick up basket and empty dishes from the SFX school office on Mondays and return the basket with food on Thursday afternoons by 3 p.m. The meals will be very much appreciated! Thank you.

In the beginning, people would bring meals to help. Maggie was able to set up a calendar of sorts on the Caring Bridge website. It was easier than having people contact the family constantly.

Fall update
October 1, 2014
By Maggie Kromm - 3 years ago

I'm downstate today and having more hyperbaric treatments that will keep me at a deeper pressure longer. I hope to get some of these treatments at McLaren soon too!

I also want to update you, I'm doing pretty well. Good days and bad moments. I've made it a mission to try to help others in our area with ALS. I have personally been in contact with the fantastic personnel at the Community Foundation in Petoskey. They used to be directly affiliated with Northern Michigan Hospital, I believe. Now we are attempting to work with McLaren in assisting patients with ALS affordable healthcare options. This will be happening soon with great support and assistance from: Shelly Budnick, Dr. Carin Nielsen, Moon Seagren, Marcia Spiegel, Maggie Kromm, Kim Wroblewski, and Deanna Beaudoin. Sorry if I missed any other instrumental names in this adventure. I am deeply touched to find out the ALS fund through the Community foundation will be named in my honor. This fund will benefit other individuals along with myself to help offset the financial cost of this disease, whether it's supplements, HBOT treatments or other medical costs associated with this disease. Specifics are being worked out now. This pleases me beyond words! As all of you know I wanted more than just me to benefit from HBOT and hyperbaric chambers. I will keep you informed on upcoming fund-raisers for this fund. Tentatively there may be a bowling fund-raiser at Northern Lights on October 17th. For more information please contact Kim Wroblewski or Deanna Beaudoin as, Medical Society Alliance members, they are doing this to raise awareness, help pay for my treatments and the community foundation fund.

Also, some of you may have heard, we sold our house! We're excited and renting first while planning next steps. Possibly building! And yes, I will be planning on having a hyperbaric chamber built in! What an awesome therapy! I'll keep all of you posted! God's not done with me yet, maybe once in a house I can begin the novel of this journey?

I pray all of you and your families are well! I will be with you in spirit! Hugs, MaryFran

Fundraising update from Kim

October 1, 2014

By Maggie Kromm - 3 years ago

Here is an update on the bowling fund-raiser. It will be October 17th from 6 to 9 pm. There is going to be a fund set up at McLaren Northern Michigan hospital foundation in MaryFran's name. It will be finalized this week. We are looking for people to sponsor a lane the night of the fund-raiser. $500 sponsorship will get you bowling for six people and advertising. If we don't sell all the lanes, then we will open bowling up for other people at a certain cost. People can also come for a cost just to have pizza and pop. We will also have a 50-50 raffle, mystery games, some door prizes and possible silent auction items. We already have a couple donors for silent or door prize items. All the money in the fund will go to people suffering from ALS as per MaryFran's request. This is how she wanted it. The foundation will help pay her costs except for medication. She wants to help the other lady in the area who also has ALS.

Fran update

October 11, 2014

By MaryFran Kolp - 3 years ago

I'm so honored and so blessed for all of the prayers …they truly have carried me…the friendships and family all you angels doing God's work, meals, setting up fundraising for the cause and helping with watching my kids. As many of you know we sold our house and are renting from our very generous friends thx Rawsons until we find something we like closer to town. As some of you may know, I have been down state this past week getting hyperbaric treatment again. They are very helpful for me. I pray all of you have a wonderful fall season! I'll be in touch soon if we don't see you at the ALS fund-raiser at the bowling alley this coming Friday!

Endless gratitude from MaryFran
By Maggie Kromm – 10/20/2014

Thank you to all for working towards "Striking out ALS." Thank you, Northern Lights, Northern Michigan Medical Society Alliance, event sponsors and donors! What an amazing event! A special thank you to Kim Wroblewski, Deanna Beaudoin and Holly O'Donnell for spearheading this event! When I said no spaghetti dinners, I didn't even dream you would do something like this. My family and Amy's family thank you!

As a PhD in Exercise Science I began research shortly after my diagnosis, after doing some research on ALS, I stopped. Too depressing… No cure, no cause, 3-5 years to live after this diagnosis. I only realized conventional treatments were not working. As a subject in a study of my own, I've selected unconventional treatments. It only makes sense that through conventional testing such as blood work and some unconventional measures we may find out what is lacking or weak, or perhaps in my case, one piece at a time halt this disease, cure this disease or extend my quality and quantity of life, God willing! See what I'm doing, much of which is NOT covered by insurance.

FIRST, I ASSEMBLED "MY MEDICAL TEAM"

- Ed Linkner, MD-Family Medicine/ Holistic Alternative medicine-Ann Arbor
- Greg Putalik MD-Family Medicine/ Holistic Alternative medicine-Harbor Springs

- Stefen Feig, DO-Family Medicine (The "Dr. House" of my team)-Santa Cruz, CA
- David Perlmutter, MD, FACN Board Certified Neurologist and internationally recognized leader in nutritional neurology-Naples, FL
- James Tenner, MD- Director of Neurology at University of Michigan
- Dee Harris- Integrated Nutritionist at the Perlmutter Medical Center-Naples, FL

WHAT ARE MARYFRAN'S SYMPTOMS?

- Muscle weakness/aches
- Muscular twitching/Fasciculations
- Fatigue
- Speech delay
- Bell's Palsy

WHAT AM I DOING TO HELP RELIEVE MY SYMPTOMS AND FIGHT ALS?

PRAYER—With a diagnosis like this you turn to God or shut him out. I have surrendered my life to him. I offer my pain and diagnosis to others in pain or going through difficult times. God is not done with me here yet. I believe I am to be part of the cure to this disease.

KETOGENIC DIET—My diet immediately changed upon my diagnosis confirmation at the Perlmutter Medical Center. No grains, NONE, only nuts & seeds, vegetables and lean meats of all sorts and a half of piece of fruit per day. No nitrates, additives aspartame or MSG. Organic foods locally grown preferred. (A special thank you to Coveyou Farms!) Due to discovered food allergies through this process, no consumption of eggs, dairy or chocolate have been added to my no consumption list.

MEDICATIONS I have opted to not take the only FDA approved medication for ALS (Reglan) as it only offers 2-3 months and can cause potential liver problems. I am taking Tamoxifen ($10 copay), Progesterone ($10 co-pay), Glutathione IV infusion ($600 monthly out of pocket).

HOMEOPATHIC REMEDIES ($6,000 paid thus far out of pocket) Cell salts, numerous tinctures for metals, parasites, environmental toxins, identified as needed by a non-approved in the USA device called an advanced thermal screening process. Adrenal capsules and Smart Silver for immune system support are also taken.

NUTRITIONAL SUPPLEMENTS ($1,800 monthly out of pocket)

- Ultra Nutrient-antioxidants and phytonutrients
- Ultimate Antiox full spectrum
- Magnesium citrate
- Low dose aspirin
- Super Ubiquinol CoQ10-enhanced mitochondrial support
- S-Acetyl Glutathione synergy
- CuraPro-antioxidant
- Neurochondria
- Inosine-building block for DNA and RNA
- Gaba
- Nrf2 Activator-Perlmutter developed/antioxidant and detoxification
- Serine
- Trehalose
- A-AKG Powder
- Nutrilite Intestiflora 7-probiotic

- Nitric acid
- Omega flax seed
- MCT oil
- Vit B12
- Vit D3
- PROmega DHEA
- BrainSustain-supports mitochondrial energy production, neurotransmitter production & cell membrane integrity.

HYPERBARIC TREATMENTS ($135 per session- over $8,000 paid thus far out of pocket)

Hyperbaric oxygen therapy, also called HBOT, is simply 100% oxygen administered to the entire body at greater than normal atmospheric pressure.

PHYSICAL & OCCUPATIONAL THERAPY Thank you to the Budnicks of Orthosport and Dr. Wroblewski's Hand Therapy of Petoskey clinic for treatments, exercises & the H wave!

REIKI AND CRANIAL SACRAL THERAPY & ACUPUNCTURE- October start

November update
By MaryFran Kolp – 11/21/2014

Hello everyone! Just wanted to give you a little update! Thus far I am doing very well. I am continuing my supplements, looking forward to a few more hyperbaric treatments, and I've also begun acupuncture and cranial sacral therapy. This has been an amazing experience and really helps me. In addition, I truly believe, diet and exercise have made a big difference in my health. I am still on a strict ketogenic diet. That means I eat no grains, but I do consume a lot of organic meats and plenty of vegetables along with many nuts and seeds without any limitations or portion sizes needed. As for what's new, Kim Wroblewski and myself are having the honor of meeting Amy Janisse, who has ALS in Indian River tomorrow. Some of the funds earned from the ALS strikeout fund-raiser were allocated to her also. We are looking forward to our meeting. In addition, The Medical Society Alliance will be adopting her family this year. They are very grateful!

Also new, we are happy to report that the Kolps are closing on a new home in Petoskey and we can't wait! It will be so nice to be close to school and town. We won't be moving in until late February or early March due to some of the renovations that will be taking place in our home. We are so blessed to have the rental opportunity of a beautiful log home this winter from Lynn and Blaine Rawson. We are very grateful.

Also, we want to thank you for all the wonderful meals we have been receiving from the organic cooking club from Julienne Tomatoes and from families personally. We are so appreciative! Well, this is just a brief update, we wish everyone a very happy and blessed Thanksgiving, and may you have a safe and restful holiday! Hugs and prayers until we meet again! Love, MaryFran

Since they lived out in the country, about twelve miles from town, they decided that they needed to move into town to be closer to the high school. Their home sold quickly, and since they had not found anything, friends of ours offered their vacant home for their use. When they finally found a home, they needed to do some renovations before they could move in. It was a great location, walking distance to the high school and centrally located. MaryFran swore that this was another divine intervention. Houses do not sell that quickly, especially out in the country where we live! The house they found was almost directly across from Petoskey High School—another blessing.

December update
By MaryFran Kolp – 12/20/2014

Merry Christmas! I just had a checkup and it appears I'm doing fine! Still weak but the ketogenic diet, supplements and treatments are working to slow or hold off some symptoms! We're so blessed this Christmas season! All the support has been such a blessing! We have no words for it! We're enjoying the rental we are in! It is a beautiful huge log home! And we have enjoyed entertaining in it this holiday season! Recently we purchased a home in Petoskey and are so looking forward to being closer to the high school for all our kids' activities. Forgive me for not sending Christmas cards this year, but we will be sending our new address in the new year! Hugs to all of you and blessings!

January update
By MaryFran Kolp – 1/9/2015

Happy New Year! One week and I'm off to Florida for 10 days, I will contact Dr. Perlmutter and his nutrition staff! I'm still on a strict ketogenic diet! Thanks to Terri Reynolds my sis in-law for all her support in cooking. Thank you everyone for your blessings and good wishes during the Christmas season. I am doing quite well. I love my medical team! Thank you Dr. Putalik, Flora Waters and Helen Durulo this month! I've added homeopathy and cranial sacral therapy and acupuncture to my routine! After an intense detoxification program, prayer and now energy work I have been blessed with making progress, positive progress! My motto remains "whatever it takes," and I don't mind hard work! Also, I'm hoping Maggie Kromm is still willing to help me document my journey, my story. I do hope it can help others and their families on their journeys. Oh, I also want to thank those of you that purchased be brave bravelets, which are bracelets that fund the cause! At bravelets.com select MaryFran whatever it takes! We were just awarded $170 for your purchases! Thank you! We're grateful it helps towards my alternative healthcare costs! Like I always say...one day at a time...it's all we have anyway! There may be many doing better but be sure some are doing worse! Treasure your gifts and use um! Hugs to all of you! Make this a new year not to forget! I am!

Heading to Florida
By MaryFran Kolp – 1/17/2015

Marie Law and I are jet setters for Florida! Blessed to visit Jim and Mary Hammond, my folks and Roger and Barb Kromm for a few weeks while thawing out and having medical follow up appointments! Megan and Genevieve and Maggie Kromm will be joining us along with my beloved hubby too! Many thanks to all who are making this possible for me! Especially, David and Maria for the condo! Looking forward to all of it! Especially the sun! I'll post updates! Enjoy the snow while we are gone!

Florida update
by MaryFran Kolp — 1/25/2015

Sunny and 70! Everyone should be here! Here's the update, I have been blessed with good weather, good friends, great accommodations and fantabulous meals by many! A special thanks to Marie and Maggie for making this all possible! They were excellent nurses on this journey! Marie would let me stay up and watch HGTV and have a glass of wine until the wee hours of the evening! Maggie made sure I was in bed at a decent hour but gave an excellent shoulder massage! She should go into business! I did have a follow-up doctor's visit with my integrative nutritionist and it was very successful. Also, a very well-respected integrated physician from Santa Cruz, California has been assisting with my case. We are doing some additional testing blood work and other stuff based on some of the new research out on ALS. Dr. Stephen Feig and Dr. David Perlmutter...let's press on for a cure! In addition, I have some new pea protein shakes and recipes to aid me in maintaining my weight! So, it will be interesting to see the results of this testing and see how the dietary changes assist me. Maggie and Genevieve and Megan arrived 2 days ago we have had fun in the sun, and plenty of shopping, and again some great meals and great laughs! I'm so glad they were able to come down and thaw out with me. I've been blessed to visit with family and friends down here including my folks, Jim and Mary Hammond, Barb and Roger Kromm, Kelly Prue! Hugs to all of you! Andy arrived today, ready to thaw out too! I'm so glad he's here! I've missed him! Thanks for holding up the fort at home! I miss you Danny! I'll see you Thursday! Good luck in your basketball game on Tuesday! We'll be watching! I'll keep all of you posted! Hugs and blessings!

Returning home from Florida
By MaryFran Kolp 1/29/2015

All good things must come to an end, so more good things can begin again! I'm heading home...going from palm trees and sun to pine trees and snow! Just sitting here on our drive upstate counting my blessings! I can't wait to see my teenagers and my friends! I missed y'all. Your words of inspiration during my time away were very much appreciated and prayers felt! It was nice to have Megan and Genevieve for a few days.

Big month for the Kolps coming up! Cleaning and getting stuff pitched and cleaned for the move into our new house at the beginning of next month! I'll keep you posted when we'll need help! Thanks Dan Cleary our contractor that sticks to schedule! We're so blessed!

Next steps regarding ALS treatment... I will be making a trip to California soon for additional testing and possible treatments. I will know more in the next few weeks. While in Florida, Marie and I discussed the possibility of a lip sync ALS fund-raiser. Upcoming treatments may be costly, so let Marie Law know if you are willing to participate in a lip sync fund-raiser to help offset cost, as again a lot of these interventions are not covered by insurance! Ohhhhh and yes, the only way Andy got me on the plane to come home was to plan spring break!! Hahaha a return to warm weather! We'll be in Fort Myers Beach over break! Part of this destination choice is I have a follow up appointment with Dr. Perlmutter then. Well I just can't end without thanking everyone that made it possible for me to thaw out and most importantly those that cared for my babies while I was away: Terri and Craig Reynolds; Carol and Carl Kolp; Kim Wroblewski, Shelley & Alan Budnick, Kim Scholl, Becky Tanis, and especially my husband... For being my rock! A special thanks to the Julienne Tomatoes cooking club members, Maggie Kromm, Lisa Leavy, Val Meyerson, Jennifer Waldvogel, Deborah Gagnon, Lynn Rawson, Deanna Beaudoin, Ann Frank, and Kim Wineman for having meals prepared for us for our return! And special thanks to, Eberharts, Ledinghams, Whitmans and cooking club members for your purchasing of these organic whole foods for my family! I know many are on the list to support through the summer! Thank you! Yes! This is part of the reason my kids are so tall!!! Thanks Julie & Tom too!!! Well time to sign off we're almost home! Love you all! Keep us in your prayers and hug your family tonight in thanks!!! What blessings we all have that we don't always acknowledge... be grateful!

FRANTABULOUS FRIENDS

Our friend Deanna Beaudoin found a book—called *Share the Care*—that helped us form a support group for MaryFran. Several of our friends read it and we decided that we could adapt it to fit MaryFran's needs. MaryFran was known for making up funny words, and she always used to say, "That is fantabulous." We decided to call our group Frantabulous Friends. The following was her entry after our initial meeting.

Share the Care meeting Success
By MaryFran Kolp 2/4/2015

I was surrounded by a group of beautiful women today that have initiated a willingness to assist me and my family in the event my health status warrants it! A special thank you to Kim Wroblewski and Maggie Kromm for hosting and facilitating this get together. These ladies discovered a book/program to assist families in caring for a loved one with an illness while not compromising their own families. It is done by sharing the load with many willing helpers. Some caregivers have big jobs, such as facilitating a monthly schedule, others a simple meal preparation and others assisting in transporting my kids, just to name a few. Being the smart, proactive, group of women I'm so blessed to be part of we kicked this process off today! If you were at the meeting I thank you, your being there means more than you'll ever know! As you saw firsthand with laughter and tears this has been a blessed journey with what I believe to be a divine purpose! I shared my ketogenic diet, talked about supplements, shots and glutothione IV pushes, along with my symptoms, acupuncture, cranial sacral therapy and Hand Therapy of Petoskey and Orthosport PT, and next steps for travel and treatment. No worries if you didn't know about the meeting or couldn't make it…you can check out the book on your own called *Share the Care* or contact Maggie Kromm, Kim Wroblewski or the SFX school office where you can check out the paperwork and share what your talents might be if you were to choose to assist if or when the time comes! It's better to be prepared up front. Those of you with other family members or friends with an illness consider this book! I pray for all with illnesses, a special prayer and blessing to my niece Dana who's experiencing some health issues, but her doctors are working hard to get her well! Please continue to keep her in your prayers too! Hugs and blessings to all my Frantabulous Friends!!!

During the meeting, she was overcome with emotion by the amount of support she was getting from her friends. We had everyone fill out forms, stating what their level of contribution would be. It included what they were good at and were willing to do. We asked for people to "captain" a week with another person. Our beginning group had eighteen captains. The captains were in-charge of getting other people to do whatever work that needed to be done. We split into groups of two to three people so that we would have to be "on" once every seven weeks or so. Other people offered to run errands, clean, bring meals, do laundry. As her illness progressed we would change our group as needed. I sent out the first schedule in May of 2015. Each schedule would be for four to six months. In the beginning, there wasn't a lot for us to do. Also, Andy did not have a traditional nine to five job, so we had to be available for evenings, nights, and weekends. As MaryFran progressed, our duties increased, and the group had to make changes and evolve. Each Friday, the captains for the next week would check in with the previous captains to see what was needed for their week. Usually, if Andy wasn't working he didn't really need us to come in to help unless he needed to run to the bank or the store or needed some much-needed "me" time.

Our group initially followed the *Share the Care* book. But we found a different way to support MaryFran that I think everyone in our group would agree worked for us. Here are some things that made our Frantabulous Friends work.

You need an organizer and implementer. This ended up being me. I will not sugarcoat this. It is a lot of work, especially toward the end. My phone blew up quite regularly with texts, emails, and calls. Fortunately, I think I was able to manage it and my family life fairly-well. I work for my husband and make my own hours. My employees knew MaryFran and were extremely understanding. My job was to send emails and updates to the group, expressing MaryFran's wishes and creating the captain schedule. I was also a captain and emotional-support person for MaryFran. I was the liaison with Andy and the kids. In retrospect, I probably took on too much, but I usually do in everything I do.

Maggie helped with coordinating meals. She set up a sign-up online (I am pretty tech savvy but not with this kind of stuff). She also found the blogging app, CaringBridge. She would also get Andy's work schedule and the kids' sport schedules and put them on a Google calendar. She was pretty much my copilot.

Even though we filled out the forms and made up binders, we did not use them like we thought we would. We decided what worked best was the captains of the week would just handle everything themselves for their week. We all liked to know that it was our week with Fran. If the three or four people didn't have coverage, then we would reach out to others in the group.

Some of the captains also decided to do specific jobs weekly. Julie would come and clean either every week or every other week. Jen and would come do baths on Tuesdays and Thursdays. Cheryl H. would come and cook special meals for Fran on Wednesdays. Others would just stop by and throw a load of laundry in or come and see if dishes needed to be put away even if they weren't "on." Usually, it was an excuse to stop by and say hi to Fran. Kim S. was our holiday-decorating extraordinaire.

Andy's sister Terri was always around to help, too. Initially, she wanted to be a captain, but we refused to put her on the list. Our reasoning was that she was already doing so much; we did not want her added on and feel like she was obligated to do more than she already was. Everyone should be so lucky to have a Terri in their life.

They pretty much had an open-door policy at the house. We had to come up with a sign system for "bad days" or days that they did not want visitors. If the green smiley face was showing, come on in. If the red sleepy face was showing, come back later. We also had a rule: if there were three people already visiting, come in and say hello, then come back later. Even though she loved a good party, the further along she progressed it was harder for her to handle a lot of noise and commotion.

By fall of 2017, we decided to increase the amount of people on each week to a minimum of three ladies. By this time, it took two people to help shower her and to help her move from place to place in the home, as she was still able to walk with help. We also needed someone to be with her at all times, especially when Andy was at work. At this point, we had our "showering" ladies, "bathroom" ladies, and "putting to bed" ladies. Having these assignments lessened the amount of people having to do her personal care. It also helped her retain some dignity by not having everyone attend to these essential duties. Since she had lost the use of her hands first, she needed help feeding, dressing, and all personal care.

By the winter of 2018, we had twenty-four active captains. These ladies were an essential part of MaryFran's care! A couple were nurses, but all were friends of MaryFran's and not all of us knew each other in the beginning. I can honestly tell you that we are now bonded for life through this journey, and there were no fighting or disagreements. We always came together to help. It wasn't always easy. But then life is never easy.

Last Stages of Moving
By MaryFran Kolp 2/18/2015

Hello Friends! Great news for the Kolps! Dana, our niece, is doing much better and back to school! We are almost done with renovations before we move in our home…and we are so excited!!! Thank you all for your prayers and blessings and your physical help!!! We have some final dates and some areas where we could use some help to get us through this, hope to be, final process!!! Movers are coming Friday, February 27th therefore, if anyone is willing to help transport/pack smaller loads on Monday, February 23rd between 11 and 1. Or Tuesday, February 24 from 12-2 or Wednesday, February 25th 11-1. Or clean Reycraft on the 26th…any or all help is appreciated!!! No pressure just if your schedule permits you to do so! Thanks everyone!!!

Moving this week
By MaryFran Kolp 2/23/2015

Thank you in advance to all of you for your help moving this week! Since it's so cold today we will focus on boxing up some things and carrying some boxes and crates from the basement up and possibly start cleaning! Since it's so cold I don't want people freezing doing multiple trips to the Petoskey house today! Having said that could some of you check for boxes and bring newspaper for packing stuff? See some of you at 11!

ShNIKE's moving is almost complete
By MaryFran Kolp 2/25/2015

What an amazing and blessed team we have had in this second or third and fourth moving process! We are almost done moving from the Reycraft home to the Petoskey house! The majority of our items have been so graciously moved! Tomorrow will be a big cleaning day at the Reycraft house. Anyone that has some time is welcome to come help. We have a few more loads to be transported. And then we will be cleaning from top to bottom the Reycraft house. Anytime between 9:30 a.m. until noon! I don't expect it will take that long! Hugs and thanks to everyone! Blessings and thanks!

Moving update
By MaryFran Kolp 2/26/2015

Great progress! Friday movers come to get the big stuff at 9am. Some cleaning and transporting some items, like plants and hamsters are needed, but no pressure if you're crazy busy…I'm just putting it out there but hope to not put anyone out! Hugs to all! I'm hanging in there! I can say certainly without the help of many I don't know how we could have done this move! Andy and I both are spinning! Thanks to all of our gracious help with sugar and whip cream and a cherry on top! Next steps, Andy may need assistance from someone or two with trucks to get a few things, like tools and such from the garage… If anyone has a truck and doesn't mind a little dirt 10- noon on Saturday, he could use your help! Please call Andy and let him know you can lend a hand!

Kolps are moved in but not yet settled

By MaryFran Kolp 3/4/2015

We can't begin to thank all of you that have made this move as smooth as possible! I must admit once moved I thought things would get easier with the house but sorting boxes, deciding what goes and what stays and where it goes has been a little crazy! The kids' social calendars have picked up momentum, just as we hoped it would! Friends in and out…we're loving every minute of it!

I must admit health wise I'm tired but who wouldn't be, even under normal circumstances!

As for medical updates…I am doing one day at a time! We are looking forward to going on spring break with family to Florida and spending time with my folks and the Collins family. The kids can't wait! After that, Andy and I will be visiting some specialists in the San Francisco Bay area in April on neurological disorders and detoxification of mitochondria! It will be interesting.

We are almost through the final stages of moving in and renovations for this phase. If you have some time or energy not compromising your own family needs we will love an hour or two to help with whatever… Carrying boxes or gifting of items to Salvation Army or the Women's Resource Center, cleaning, organizing… Will gladly take an hour or two or come have tea! Hugs to all of you and again thank you for your prayers and support!

During this time, I found out that another young woman in our area was dealing with ALS. MaryFran wanted to visit her. We set up a meeting and MaryFran asked me if I would drive her to meet her, as she lived about forty-five minutes away. The young woman was in her early thirties and had a young son. She unfortunately did not have as much help as we did. She was in fairly-advanced stages and could barely speak. It was very sobering for MaryFran to see and the drive back home was terrible.

MaryFran kept saying, "I cannot believe I'm going to end up like that." It was one of the first times in my life when I honestly did not know what I could say to her. I just told her that she was going to be trying different treatments that this other lady had not tried, and that hopefully she would not end up like that. It took everything I could do in my power not to break down and cry uncontrollably. I kept thinking, *this cannot be possible*. She asked me if I thought she should try alternative treatments. I told her that if I were in her shoes and they told me I had to drink horse pee, I would. It became a joke between us. Unfortunately, this young lady died on January 14, 2018.

My first fall but humorous story
By MaryFran Kolp 3/13/2015

I just felt I had to share the story. Yes, I had my official first fall... But was it really a fall because of ALS? On my way to La Dolce Vita, the best salon in town in my opinion, as the ladies at the salon have really taken care of me and offered treatments to keep me going since my diagnosis! On with the story... I was getting ready to go for a pedicure. When I drove my car and parked I had contemplated in the middle of March with snow banks still piled high in Northern Michigan whether I should hurdle the snow bank in flip flops, or walk around and put money in the meter that way? I proceeded to hurdle the snowbank wiped out on my caboose and had re-created the reenactment of Ralphie from the Christmas story movie with my glasses all plugged up with snow! So, a lesson learned...don't hurdle snow banks in flip flops!!!

Moving update
By MaryFran Kolp 3/13/2015

We are officially moved in! New carpet is due to arrive next week. Then we're taking a break, to do taxes and start saving to do more with the house later this year! We absolutely love our kitchen! Most of our painting is complete due to "two chicks and a stick" Julie Izzard and Lynn Rawson are amazing painters they don't even tape off! We are really enjoying the house, especially its location! It seems like weeks ago when we were trying to move all of our belongings in - 13 to - 23 degree weather. With snow blowing sideways! And dust still flying at our new destination to be called home due to renovations!

To top it off…We also survived moving without Andy's truck due to his third accident all of which he wasn't even near his truck when a semi took the whole side of his vehicle out! While he was enjoying a coffee at North Perks! So, there we were moving without our truck. But, due to many of you and your vehicles we were successful and getting everything moved over! We still can't believe all of the help and support not one time not even 2 times but assisting us in moving 3 times all within a 6 month time period! Crazy! Lastly, life continues to happen as the heat has gone out twice in our new house. Luckily, I think the problem is now fixed! Maybe we're destined to be cold this winter! Thanks again for stepping up and all your help, moving, painting, cooking, meals, support, cleaning, sorting, putting my closet together and love! Hugs and blessings to all of you!

Spring is in the air
By MaryFran Kolp 3/20/2015

I am sitting at my new counter, in my new kitchen, with my old dog counting my blessings! So many of you, and others, have just stepped up or stepped in and just did what needed to be done to get this house and my family in working order. It was done with love and true gratitude. We truly don't deserve this beyond spectacular help and treatment! Your prayers, support and actions have fed our bodies and souls. Thank YOU, no-matter how much or how little you feel you've done, it's been huge to us!

Medical update...Yesterday, I had an appointment with, my local physician Dr. Greg Putalik. He has been very supportive of me and in working with the groups of physicians and health professionals contributing their knowledge to my case! My appointment went well! I haven't progressed. Not better but not worse. I am stable. Also, I've put on 4 lbs. That's good for me! Thanks Cheryl Hooley to tastefully increasing the fat and calories in my diet! Or maybe it's weight gain by osmosis! I've been frequenting Julienne Tomatoes picking up pecan rolls for our helpers at the house!

Now that I am in a stable state I have decided to push forward with alternative treatments. We can't beat this wondering when it's going to progress and how...therefore, no cause no cure...press on. Andy and I will be leaving for the San Francisco bay area in late April. I will be seeing and receiving treatment from 3 specialists. Dr. Stephen Feig, D.O., Dr. Lin, D.O. and Dr. Beth McDougal, D.O. Dr. Feig has been my sounding board and has prepared me with supplements, referrals and support while preparing for my visit with Dr. Perlmutter in Naples. If you haven't checked out the book "The Grain Brain" written by Dr. David Perlmutter, do so...dementia, Alzheimer's, ADD... Neurological disorders... Something in there for all of us or our families. Good news for Dr. Perlmutter he's retiring. Happy for him as he will be retired but still working in the field of neurology rumor has it, ALS research! I will be working closely with Dr. Feig and some of his colleagues. Dr. Lin, DO is a structural wizard and uses a lot of energy work. Also, Dr. Beth McDougal, DO her emphasis is mitochondrial detoxification. I will be going for an evaluation and a treatment. I have been continuing with acupuncture and cranial sacral therapy with Helen Diriglio at Root Health these past few months. She has assisted my body in amazing energy movement work. I highly recommend her. Also, I have been working with Flora Waters utilizing homeopathic remedies to provide support for my systems and organs where needed. I too am so grateful for the hand, wrist and shoulder therapy from Dr. Fred Wroblewski's Hand Therapy of Petoskey and PT support from the Budnicks at Orthosport. Some may think I'm a little crazy doing all this alternative support. I am crazy, but it's working, helping anyway…traditional medicine literature regarding ALS doesn't impress me yet. Time will tell! As for hyperbaric oxygen treatments, I'll get back to them, but for now financially I have selected to stay local and focus on acupuncture/cranial sacral therapy. I miss hyperbaric but with moving and traveling with Megan to her AAU tournaments for volleyball… I haven't been able to get downstate to fit them in. As for immediate next steps, thanks to the assistance of Marie Law I am in the process of doing voice recordings in the event disease progression expedites and I can no longer yell at my children Ha-ha! I hope I don't need this for a long time but its best to over prepare! I apologize this is pretty long-winded but wanted to bring all of you up to speed. Your continued prayers are felt and appreciated! More than you'll ever know! Happy spring!!!

Happy Easter to all!
By MaryFran Kolp 4/4/2015

I hope all of you had a great spring break and Holy Week! Happy Easter to all of you! We had a fabulous break in Fort Myers Florida! We were blessed to hang with some of our friends and family over break! My folks, the Collins family, Law and Hammond families, the Kromms, the Kirbys, Burnhams, Jakeways, O'learys and new friends Rex and Nan!!! With sand on our toes, great food and beverage and gorgeous weather & great socializing… What a blessed blast! It felt so good to thaw out! I pray too you had a wonderful Easter celebration wherever you may be! I so enjoyed the warm weather! I attempted to pack some warmth and sunshine in my suitcase for home! We'll see what happens!

Our next journey is a visit to Mill Valley, California to see specialists in April! We're still working on this illness day by day! We will be staying part of the time with the Collins family in between appointments, we look forward to some positive direction from the docs in California! I had a lesson in HOPE watching March madness basketball…Anyone watch the final four Kentucky Wisconsin game? Kentucky was a stacked team 38-0 this season…. But once again I was reminded nothing is impossible… Wisconsin beat Kentucky… And Wisconsin will be playing in the national championship game against Duke! With will power and hard work…you always have a shot! Nothing is impossible is it? I'll remember this in my daily struggles! I hope you will too! Happy Easter! May you appreciate what our Lord has given you!!! Always remember you are very special and more than enough… You are made in his image, never underestimate the power in that alone!

What's MaryFran really feeling
By MaryFran Kolp 4/5/2015

I had hoped the sunshine and warmth I packed in my suitcase would have made it at least 24 hours to Northern Michigan Ha-ha! Mother nature had other plans as I watch the snowflakes fall on the bushes in our backyard! As for this post I've been texted and emailed by many of you…how am I REALLY doing? So, I thought I would share a little more, it too will help me work through my answers to this question. Like Robin Roberts says, "everybody's got something!" This journey with ALS has shown me I am loved more than I deserve by those around me, my family, friends, church and community, even friends from the past, high school and college have contacted me and we've caught up and reconnected. This has been a pretty incredible experience! I usually don't mind being the center of attention, but this has been a different experience. I'm not sure if it is fear that I'm going to wear out the help I have? Or that I'm going to really need a lot of help in the future? Or If I beat this disease people will question whether I had it at all. I do believe this journey has a lesson in it. Don't think I'm not frightened from time to time I asked why me? Why ALS? In response, Why not me? I'm not sure if I'm supposed to show people how to live? Or how to die? There are a ton of emotions and questions, as you can imagine, that go along with this. That now I'm forced to face. Some days I feel like I can beat this, hands down! Other days, I think about getting my voice digitalized because I may lose it... So like Marie Law says, "Plan for the worst and hope for the best!" I think about writing letters to my husband and children and friends if I proceed to the other side before they do. And then there's grandchildren and great-grand babies. I will be with all of them but differently! The thought makes me sad to not be here, if that's what God wills, but if it is, I must trust, and you should too.

I have to say this Holy Week and Easter season has been different from others for me. I put myself in Jesus' shoes in the garden of Gethsemane. What a deep faith but torment he must have felt. No words can explain his journey. While myself being sick and knowing what I might die from and the potential grueling end process, it is scary, but I BELIEVE in the after physical life. I have too!!! If I'm made in God's image this can't be it. But I do think we've seen glimpses of it here on earth. A sunset, a new born child, first steps, making love with your spouse after a nice glass of wine by the fire place, smiles, Christmas morning in a child's eyes, new carpet...a gourmet kitchen finished... ha, ha, ha, ha, ...don't you agree? Jesus died a gruesome death for us all. I offer up my suffering to others that are sick, poor, lonely, or in pain or contemplating abortion. I think, children's prayers are heard first... But you move up on the list when sick too. So, if you need a prayer please let me know!

As for my actual pain now, it's limited to cramping of muscles and fear of the unknown. My muscles and their relationship with my nerves are crazy. I often feel jittery. I do have extensive weakness in my left arm...all stemming from a weakness in my neck. Lifting a 4 oz. glass feels like a gallon of milk to me. Also, it's difficult to lift my left arm over my head. Through energy work I have tried to remain positive and limit weakness if not stop its progression. So, if my hair looks challenged, it's because I couldn't lift my arms to do it or I have an upcoming appointment at La Dolce Vita, with Chanin, the owner that has donated her service to me to help keep up my hair! So, since I've been ill many are keeping me looking good! I tire easily. I just can't do it all anymore. I almost turned old overnight. Move slow, eat slow, takes forever to cook and clean and move! Lesson learned... be patient with old people and the ill. They don't move slow or act cranky to cheese you off. They, like me, just can't move and adjust like they used too!

These are some of my thoughts from the heart. Melody Collins sent me a great quote I thought I'd share with you. Ignatius says "pray as if God will take care of it all; act as if it's all up to you!" I love you all as many of you had asked what's she really feeling...well here's a glimpse!

What's MaryFran doing to combat this disease
By MaryFran Kolp 4/11/2015

First, daily I count my blessings! Seriously, although tired, my skin looks great, my waist line because of my ketogenic diet is just fine. My husband's healthy, and is working, we have insurance, my kids are healthy and doing great in school and on the courts! My parents and in-laws are healthy. I'm so blessed by friends, good friends…love you when you're feeling great or not feeling so great! Those are the keepers, they never let me down! Three things I'm doing right now that I feel is instrumental to my wellness. Prayer and meditation, acupuncture and cranial sacral therapy, and lastly homeopathies and supplements. Prayer and meditation especially when using my electrical stimulation machine. This machine can be set for certain frequencies to stimulate or calm my muscle and nerve connections. Although not approved by the FDA, this device is used for many medical purposes abroad! I don't mind it and sleep with the electrodes on nightly!

The second thing, I have selected to accept the positive energy work received through acupuncture and cranial sacral therapy. I begin face up and needles, thinner than a hair are placed in certain specific locations, this aids in balancing my chakras, medians, energy systems. The needles do not hurt and often I don't even feel them there, unless there is an energy block sometimes you can feel a little discomfort, but it's tolerable because I know it's helping my body help itself! The cranial sacral experience is one I've never previously experienced. The trained professional cradles your head and neck in one hand and your sacrum in the other. Slight movements shift the fluid in the brain and spine and the bones and muscles to be aligned for optimal performance. During this process, I have experienced a light feeling. Often with my eyes closed I see an array of colors and I'm told this is a good thing! Lastly, but not least, the supplements I take are plant based and provide a support for all my systems. Especially being on a ketogenic diet (no grains or starches or sugars of any kind) I am on supplements to support my mitochondria. Mitochondria are the power houses of our cells for energy production and mine are on overload, this may be sparing the deterioration of my muscle and nerves. For now, I administer a B12 shot daily to myself, and take from 24 to 15 capsules 3 times per day of vitamins, minerals, mitochondrial enhancers, enzymes, etc. Lastly, I take homeopathic remedies also 3 times per day. These are natural medicines composed of minute doses of plant, mineral and animal substances that stimulate the body's immune system. When these substances are given in very small safe doses they bring about a healing reaction. Homeopathic medicines are relatively inexpensive without side effects and completely safe to use. Unlike conventional medicine, homeopathic medicines work with the body to defend itself and do not inhibit the natural healing process.

As most of you know I will be leaving for California to see some specialists next week regarding my condition. There are some new treatments to enhance mitochondrial efficiency, to provide detoxification of symptoms so they can work optimally and again having someone looking at me from a structural standpoint assessing my actual bone structure and alignment. Nevertheless, this is going to be an enlightening experience. I will keep you tuned as I learn more! Blessings of warmth and goodness to all of you!

Arrived safely in Reno
By MaryFran Kolp 4/20/2015

Andy and I arrived last evening in Reno! Our flights were uneventful. That's a good thing. As I looked about the plane the lady next to me was reading, Robin Roberts book, "Everybody's Got Something" I've quoted before in these CaringBridge blogs and the lady in front of me was reading on "Angels! Divine Interventions for Sure!" While I'm reading Mitch Albom's "Tuesdays with Morrie" good book if you haven't read it. I am reading it not because I'm a glutton for punishment, but I offered to speak to the Honors English classes at Petoskey high when I return from California. Compare and contrast some things in the book and sharing my story. Danny is in one of the classes and they are reading this book. FYI Danny's teacher and counselor did discuss in advance with us Danny's reading this. Dan and I talked about it and he wants to read it. I thank his teacher for her compassion. In a nut shell, and I'm living this...the premise of the book is that you really don't begin to live until you find out you may die!

This morning we woke up to a beautiful view with our very generous hosts and friends, Jeff and Melody Collins! We are staying with them until we head to Mill Valley, CA on Tuesday where my appointments with specialists will begin.

Although exhausted yesterday, I feel great today! I do wonder if the altitude has anything to do with this? We are staying at 6700 ft above sea level. My muscle twitching subsided. I'm curious to see how I do on our hike this afternoon! My next adventure may be looking into ALS at altitude! I was blessed to watch Kira at a volleyball tournament in Reno this morning! She did well and the girls on her team are very kind! The tournament was huge and very impressive! Over 80 teams and it's Monday! Great day so far! I was able to type this in between games!

Meeting with the first physician specialist
By MaryFran Kolp 4/22/2015

What came first...the chicken or the egg? God only knows... doesn't She! Ha-ha I had an interesting meeting with Dr. Linn this morning. He is a fabulous physician and in tune with his work. I have never had an experience like this! Andy was with me and Dr. Linn assessed me and was right on with his findings! He identified left body weakness, predominantly upper quadrants along with neck and upper back and left ear challenges, including some sinus and lung drainage/blockage issues. With a few adjustments and further evaluation, I was referred to a biological holistic dentist to receive an evaluation and an ozone treatment! I see him tomorrow. A trigger for my neuromuscular symptoms may be attributed to a bacterial growth of some sort beginning in my teeth and gums, either from a crack, or a carryover from a previous illness or virus that manifested in what now has resulted in serious symptoms. (Hence the reason for the chicken and the egg lead in)! Some research findings have shown increased incidence in ALS symptoms when root canals have been performed. I have not had a root canal, but I have had a composite cap put on a molar in my lower left jaw. I will find out more tomorrow morning after further evaluation. In addition, I have been put on some more supplements, activated charcoal and Wobenzym, a dietary supplement used to support aches and pains from joints while detoxifying and ACS spray which kills bacteria. Lastly, and most importantly it was recommended my cocktail of choice should be an organic tequila, named Fortelezza! I'll let you know how this treatment goes later!!! Hugs to you all! Keep the prayers coming!

Second day of doctors' visits
By MaryFran Kolp 4/23/2015

Another interesting day! This morning we met with Dr. Brian Smith. Holistic Biological dentist in Mill Valley. Studied in the Seattle area and his area of expertise is oral systemic balance with mouth and autonomic dysfunction and TMJ disorders. It appears my breathing and tongue and teeth configuration may be compromised, has been for years and I've also had TMJ for years. This may be contributing to my ALS symptoms. I will know more on Monday. I will have 2 important and clarifying appointments then! It appears I will be receiving ozone treatments this next week as well. Thanks for your prayers! All has been positive! I'm learning so much! Hugs to all of you!

Sunday morning rituals

By MaryFran Kolp 4/26/2015

I'm still in California, looking forward to meeting with some specialists, tomorrow afternoon! Melody Collins will be escorting me on this trip! I've missed her, and it will be nice to have some Mel-Fran time! This morning I went to Mass in Truckee, CA. It was a beautiful church with the mountain lodge motif beautiful! We began the service singing…sing to the mountains… It had a much different impact on me being in the mountains than at home. Today was Good Shepherd Sunday… We are reminded… whatever's going on in our lives, whether it be a celebration or deep sorrow….Jesus, our unconditional loving Savior has our backs!!! Then during the Eucharistic Prayer, we were blessed to hear the priest, with an excellent voice, sing our Eucharistic Prayer in a Capella! Icing on the cake. It was a beautiful morning and I lit some candles for those in need of prayer! Prayers are welcome! Pray for the doctors meeting with us tomorrow! God bless each of you and your families! I'll post again tomorrow! Mel and I are on the veranda sharing some spirits!

Doctor's visits California style

By MaryFran Kolp 4/27/2015

Melody and I begin our day in Mill Valley at the Clear Center of Health where we met with Dr. Stephan Feig. He has been a lead consultant on my case since my diagnosis. During my appointment with Dr. Feig, he did a physical exam and did update my supplements and reviewed my blood lab results. Then we met with Dr. Beth McDougal. She is an MD utilizing many forms of testing and support in her practice including Integrated approaches, energy work and body balancing techniques. For every question I had answered today 2 or 3 more questions were created. It appears, as suspected, this is a complex issue. Toxicity issues were identified in the testing with Dr. McDougal along with structural issues with my neck and spine. In addition, increased bacteria may be a contributing culprit. To fight the bacteria, I will be getting what are called ozone injections in my jaw in the next few days to see if there is a change in my symptoms. Let's hope their are for the good! In addition, I will be getting some IV treatments for nutritional support and detoxification. These injections could potentially make me sick before I get better. But to get better that is my goal so, I will do whatever it takes. These treatments are not all new, many have been used in Europe and other countries well before being accepted here. In California many things are happening with holistic health and positive results occurring. Since traditional medicine hasn't found a cause, much less a cure for ALS nor have the pharmaceutical companies developed a pill or injection… Who's to say…unlayering my symptoms, one at a time won't end in a positive result or a cure for me…and a starting point for many others to come. Like I said I believe ALS stands for "a lot of symptoms" I don't have any answers yet, and may never have all the answers, but I have a direction for treatment… And moving forward is my goal! I'm grateful for all my doctors and specialists. Thank you for praying for them. Initial treatments begin tomorrow! I'll keep you posted!

Asking for prayers for a friend
By MaryFran Kolp 4/28/2015

You have prayed for me and my family and doctors, I regret to ask for one more. Many of you know our neighbors from the cottage Tom and Pat Terry, their daughter-in-law Lisa Terry a very kind soul, beautiful Mom, wife and a physician herself had a heart attack and collapsed downstate and they're asking for many prayers. All of you have carried me through and I'm hoping that you can forward some prayers to the Terry family and especially Lisa!

Fran update from Mill Valley
By MaryFran Kolp 4/30/2015

I am blessed to be in a beautiful area, warm and full of sunshine, receiving excellent care. I had to smile when updating Andy on my CaringBridge site when voice texting my phone picked up that I was saying "curing" bridge instead. I do hope this to be true! My first appointment of the day yesterday included a manipulation and structural treatment of my spine and my neck. This was a very beneficial treatment. I've been given exercises to lengthen my neck and spine that I will add to my regime to get well. It appears I have some structural issues that may be contributing to my ALS symptoms. These could be from numerous causes accidents, athletics, etc. Next, we visited a biological dentist, Dr. Brian Smith that gave me four ozone shots in my jaw area. The ozone shots are given to kill any bacteria that has developed in cavitations in the area where my wisdom teeth were before I had them removed in my early 20's…just a few years ago. Ha-ha! In conjunction with bacteria build up, being very sick in winter of 2013 for a 3-4 month time period my immune system couldn't keep up. Therefore, causing a potential perfect storm. The shots were a little uncomfortable but then a brief numbness, relief and a crackling sound in my left ear and jaw resulted. Shortly after the ozone shots, I did experience a decreased pressure in my head and neck, and although still weak the fasciculations subsided in my muscles, Today, some of these symptoms have reappeared however not to their original extent. Which again indicates this is a multifaceted complex issue. Following my ozone treatments, we were off to the Clear Center of Health in Mill Valley where I received a personalized nutritional IV. It appears as if I was depleted in some nutrients and cell salts therefore an IV was given for support. This was pretty relaxing actually, the cocktail had magnesium in it which made me sleepy. So, I got a great nap in the afternoon. After my IV appointment, Melody and I witnessed a bank hold up! Seriously, cops had gunman at the entrances. Quite an eventful afternoon! We didn't stick around to see what resulted, but it appears no one was hurt! All kinds of activities going on! Lastly, I have two additional IV treatments scheduled, and two additional treatments scheduled with Dr. Lin for structural manipulation. Finally, I will have another round of ozone treatments on Monday. After all of this and some supplement changes it appears I will be home in a week or so. I can't wait to see everyone! Then it appears I will be coming back to this area in 6-8 weeks for follow up treatments and evaluation. Please keep praying! So many are in need of them! Special prayers for Lisa Terry, Darby Walker and Tim Kulman and their families!

Preparing for my last round of visits in Mill Valley before I come home for awhile
By MaryFran Kolp 5/3/2015

It's Sunday evening and we were blessed with a wonderful weekend! I was able to watch Kira Collins and her volleyball team in a great tournament! The girls were very impressive! They made it to quarter finals in the final pool and unfortunately came up short. They had a great day! I was so proud to watch and be there. It was a great weekend! The next few days are going to be crazy busy until I fly home on Wednesday! I have another round of ozone-shots in the morning and IV treatments in the afternoon! The IV cocktail contains vitamin B 6, B12, magnesium, vitamin C, homeopathies of a variety. I have received 2 so far, each IV takes approximately 45 minutes to administer. Just enough time for Melody to do some shopping downtown! Then on Tuesday

I've been asked to do a 3D x-ray of my jaw and spine. So that will be done, then lastly, this visit, I will meet with Dr. Linn for a structural adjustment and energy work. Since it will be Cinco de Mayo, I will be taking organic margarita mix and organic tequila to my last appointment! Mel, Dr. Linn and I will toast...to a great cocktail!!! Ha-ha! Then Wednesday I begin my journey home flying most of the day! I will miss my home away from home here in California, but I'll be back soon. I have been given hope here! I feel like I'm on a pathway to healing but I still have a lot of work and healing to do. A lot is still unknown. I'm up for the fight, with all of your prayers and support! The Lord knows, your prayers and divine interventions have taken me this far! Thank you!

Thoughts to share from California
By MaryFran Kolp 5/4/2015

I like that saying by Ralph Waldo Emerson...Do not go where the path may lead, go instead where there is no path...and leave a trail. This is my intention. This has been and will continue to be an interesting journey! I still have a long way to go. But, like my doctors have said and Mary Hramic-Hoffman shared with me... our bodies are amazing and have the divine ability to heal itself, especially when given the support needed to do so! Our bodies and souls combined are a remarkable "machine" for lack of a better term. It's also, interesting that I would be given a diagnosis of ALS in which modern medicine has, no cause, no cure and therefore I'll add no treatment! Maybe it takes something like ALS to move the medical community and their thought processes to entertain alternative care! Diet, energy work, structural and visceral care along with ALS is complex, it's quite honestly a "son of a gun!" And I'll tell you this, a pill created by any pharmaceutical company isn't the answer and won't cure this! Another interesting observation, this entire visit to California, I have had the option

of organic, grass fed, free range non-GMO food options everywhere and not a waitress has looked at me suspicious or like I
was from another planet when ordering food to accommodate
my ketogenic dietary needs! The Midwest has a lot of catching
up to do in this area! I'm talking fast food to deli's to expensive
restaurants...crazy everyone is on board in the Mill Valley and
Corte Madera areas!! Just a few thoughts to share today. This
morning I had some more ozone treatments and I have the 3D
x-rays to determine if I have some dental cavitations contributing
to my symptoms tomorrow. I also had a nutritional IV today, and
as usual I took my supplements, those with food, those before
meals, those away from food and homeopathies and probiotics,
etc. I'm looking forward to returning home to see everyone! Just
a few scattered thoughts I thought I'd share while in Cali!!!

Trip to Cali summary

Journal entry by MaryFran Kolp — 5/6/2015

I have been gone for 3 weeks, enjoying my time with the Collins
family, especially my one-on-one time 24/7 with Melody! Andy
had to return home to tend to our children and get back to work to
pay for all of this. Therefore, Melody, with support from Jeff was
with me. She was a great help and wore many hats during my
journey...friend, counselor, nurse, secretary, chauffeur, advocate,
financial provider, hair stylist, chef, shopping advisor, etc. and
she's still talking to me! I'm still not sure if we did more laughing
or crying, but it was all good! Great in fact! Priceless memories!
A lot has happened, between treatments, appointments, shots,
manipulations, consults with doctors and dentists who think
outside the box! As for asking the hard questions, Mel helped me
with this too. Do I have ALS or something else? Recall, I received
this diagnosis and confirmation last July from respectable and
well-practiced neurologists at U of M and in Naples, Florida.

Whatever I have can we fix it? Out of the 4 specialists I saw in California, 2 are not sold on the ALS diagnosis, or think we can tackle what I have based on their evaluation of me at this time. The other 2 are not sure. Time and further treatment will tell. Alternative practitioners do not like, nor do they use "labels" in their practice like ALS. They assess a person by lab tests, blood, urine, feces, saliva, energy, physical examination, discussion with the patient, then treat each symptom or imbalance one at a time or in small groupings, then they see the body's response (mind, body, soul) and adjust protocol based on how the body responds. Nevertheless, it has been an expensive adventure. Much of what I'm doing is not covered by insurance! I don't share this to solicit funds. Simply a stated fact, we blew through close to $15,000 in 3 weeks including flight, lodging when not at Collins, food, treatments, doctor and treatment fees and consults. This is not a poor woman's disease. And the taxes and office rental fees these practitioners in California pay are crazy outrageous and obviously the tab is paid by the consumer like here! All just to get well! Thank God for the fund set aside for medical expenses. I have used it for treatments here and at home and I'm so grateful for it. I hope to use this fund for some help with medical expenses expected in June when I have to return for some follow up treatments. So, I want to thank once again those that contributed to that fund. Along with physician and specialist visits, Melody and I covered a lot of area exploring and having fun in Corte Madera, Mill Valley and my favorite Sausalito! All located in close proximity, tucked in the northern mountains of Cali! Corte Madera, cute town and two restaurants to mention that were our favorites, when not eating at whole foods, the Café Verde and the Blue Barn, great organic high quality and delicious food! Mill Valley had quaint shops and great atmosphere! They even had an organic fast food burger joint! Sausalito, love the hills and the bay and the view! We even had a few days, with light fog so we could see San Francisco across the bay. And, there is a great organic chocolate shop "Pick Me Up Chocolate" and a crystal shop with all kinds of interesting things! We even spent some time in old town Sacramento! Had great Mexican food on Cinco de Mayo! Weekends I was blessed to stay at the Collins Compound, in Truckee, CA. By Lake Tahoe! What a beautiful home! They too have some wonderful friends I met too! Jeff, Mel and Hunter and Kira are doing great! I'm so happy for them and grateful they shared their home and the surrounding area with me! It's a spectacular part of our country! Now back home I so missed my Andy and Danny and Megan! It's great to be back with them! Tomorrow we're off to the Grand Rapids-Holland area for AAU basketball tournaments for both kids! I'm looking forward to watching! Then somehow, I hope to make my Godson Ethan Reed's first communion! A busy weekend in store...One last note, and an important one I think. I have had a few people tell me with their gift of time, talent or treasure and from many of you all three T's...that if the shoe was on the other foot or roles reversed, I would be one of the first in line to help. This is true. But, I have to let those of you helping know, your gifts, I believe given by God, no matter how much or little you feel you've helped me, and my family have not gone unnoticed. I have learned too with this neuromuscular disorder, I had to receive help, and it killed me not to send a thank you at every turn or buy gifts of thanks for you. I had to receive, accept and be grateful. I do not take one action for granted! Never will. I have offered my illness up for those that have helped me...that means YOU, my family, and those hurting, sick, and those that have lost hope. Don't underestimate the gifts you've given us and others, trust me you'll reap what you sow! Being an angel of God and doing work on his behalf here on earth isn't always easy, but priceless in the eyes of Heaven! I don't plan on giving up hope to be well, it may take a while and may get worse before it gets better! I hope to inspire others that feel hopeless in whatever their "poison" hope to fight! Nothing is beyond the reach of determination, if you just believe and trust! Love you all! Thanks for reading and sharing in my journey!

Thoughts after this weekend home after 3 weeks of treatment
Journal entry by MaryFran Kolp — 5/10/2015

I was able to reconnect with old Grand Valley friends during Danny and Megan's AAU basketball tournaments this past weekend. What a treat connecting with other "old Laker athletes" and now all of us watching our children playing against each other in this tournament! Specifically, Tyler Davis (Mike Davis, Andy's best buddy and roommate and team mate in college) Mike's son and Danny played each other! What a rush watching the boys play! Congrats Tyler, their team won the tournament! It was a great organized chaotic weekend! Danny played an AAU tournament in Holland and Megan had a AAU tournament in Caledonia! Andy had to work so I drove back and forth watching the kid's games. Both kids played well! Won some and lost some. After Danny's team was done, he was asked to play in another tournament in Lansing on Sunday. Danny was able to catch a ride to Lansing as I needed to stay with Megan while she finished up in Caledonia. Then we drove to get Danny and drove home! So, for a Mom gone for 3 weeks this was the best Mother's day gift! Watching both of my kids playing a game I love! How blessed I am!

Speaking of this, as I watch my children, now young adults, I'm inspired by them. I believe looking back, I will do the best I can in defeating what I have because of what I learned in athletics. Being competitive, wanting to win and doing whatever it took as a team and an individual to succeed! Up until Kindergarten or first grade, offering awards to all for participation may be a good thing. But life isn't about everyone getting a gold star. Competition and giving credit where credit is due is a good thing it teaches us many things. How to win whatever the battle, how to lose and learn and competition helps you find and polish your gifts! For example, my kids, like Andy and I, were gifted with some skills for athletics. This is our vehicle for big life lessons, others it's band, voice, robotics, debate, etc. We need to feed and fine tune those God given gifts! These competitive experiences prepare us for the challenges we encounter in life. As for my health status after being home, I have a new revised batch of supplements and homeopathies I'm taking. Also, I will continue some traction exercises I've been given to do. I will continue acupuncture and cranial sacral therapy too here at home. And, some IV home treatments as well. Then I will prepare to return to California for another round of treatments, hopefully having my kids go with me once they are out of school in June!

Tyler Davis and Danny Kolp

Journal entry by MaryFran Kolp — 5/12/2015

Danny shooting 2 over Tyler Davis!

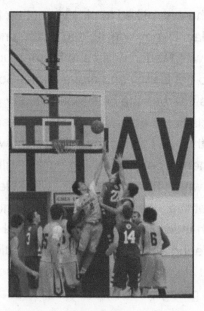

Megan and Mike Davis

Journal entry by MaryFran Kolp — 5/12/2015

Andy's best friend in college

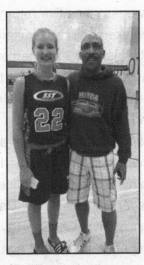

Grand Valley Laker Alumni

Journal entry by MaryFran Kolp — 5/12/2015

Great connecting with old friends again!

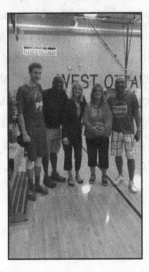

Just some thoughts

Journal entry by MaryFran Kolp — 5/16/2015

By MaryFran Kolp - 2 years ago

It's been a crazy few weeks since I've returned home from California! This past weekend alone, I traveled with Danny to Kalamazoo for an AAU basketball tournament! Because I wanted to attend our school auction, my Dad came to Kalamazoo the second day of the tournament, along with Grandpa Carl to hang with Danny. Danny and his teammates won the tournament undefeated this weekend! Danny also won an outstanding player award for the tournament. As I drove home from Kalamazoo after leaving Danny to his Granddad's house, I thought a lot about those on my prayer list: Lisa Terry, Darby Walker, Carl Vanderwall, Tim Kulman, Olivia Carlson, my children, husband and all our family members and friends! Again, I had 4 hours in the car to pray and listen to Christian Radio! Here's a challenge for you…if you haven't listened to a Christian radio station in a while, I encourage you when you're feeling a little down, put it on and listen to the words of the songs played! Inspiration and hope are loaded in the lyrics! No sexual lyrics about bumping and grinding! I'm also reminded there's something bigger than us listening to Christian radio! Try it! Trust me! You won't be sorry!

Our school auction was a great success! Dan Cleary and Katie Tarachas and their team did a great job! I too was honored along with Liz Molosky with the Crusader Award! A complete surprise and honor! Also, It was great to see friends and parishioners all dressed up and catching up on the latest at this wonderful event! A great weekend and beautiful weather too! How blessed we are!

Great gift upon my return from California appointments
Journal entry by MaryFran Kolp — 5/17/2015

Upon my return from California I was greeted by great friends,
Lynn Rawson, Julie Izzard and Deanna Beaudoin! How nice to
see my friends I missed so much! But that was only the beginning...Julie Izzard, Terri Reynolds, Kim Scholl and Dave Skop
did an HGTV job on my laundry room! My "Tiffany" inspired
laundry room is amazing! It's clean, painted, organized with bins
and shelves and decked out with Florida pictures of our kids! I
couldn't believe it. I'll post pictures! What a priceless gift! The
laundry room was so skanky before, now one of my favorite
rooms! I don't even mind doing laundry! That wasn't the only
surprise, Lynn Rawson, Jennifer Buck, Julie Izzard cleaned
my windows and blinds and planted flowers in my front pots to
greet me!!! And, a special thanks to my Dad for bringing up my
living room couch and thanks Ralph Guthrie for transporting and
hanging my mirror! I'm so crazy grateful, I don't even know how
to thank these ladies and gentlemen for all of their help and hard
work! Special blessings being sent your way! I do hope you had
some FUN!!!

Frannie update and family happenings
Journal entry by MaryFran Kolp — 5/30/2015

A lot has happened for the Kolps these last few weeks! Danny
has been blessed with being asked to play with the parallel 45
south team after his parallel 45 north season completed. The
past two weekends we've been in Kalamazoo and Mt. Pleasant,
undefeated and champions both weekends! So proud of this
group of talented boys! Wish them luck in Lansing this weekend! We also had an 8th grade graduation! Megan is officially a
high schooler! She's so ready! I'm not sure Andy and I are! Meg

is still enjoying her AAU basketball season and simultaneously has started volleyball training as well. This summer looks to be packed with activity! We wouldn't want it any other way! We are aware these high school years are short and go by very fast so we're maximizing every minute of this time!

Regarding my health, I'm stable. Not better but not worse. This I like to think is a good thing! We have begun my help from my Frantabulous Friends (who thought up that name anyway?) where a leadership team will help me and my family where we may need help or assistance. I'm so very grateful to all these helpers. Especially, Kim Wroblewski and Maggie Kromm for leading this endeavor! I hope to not require too much time at this point! Pray never!!! Nevertheless, thank you for all you've done and are willing to do to help me and my family.

As some of you know I had a very positive experience in California with my medical treatment received there. Therefore, I am planning on returning for round 2 beginning June 11th. I will be out there for about a week. I am grateful and thankful for Maggie Kromm and her kids who will be flying out there with me, and Robin Corrington who will be assisting me and will help get me back. Some of the treatments I will be receiving will be a little more intense than last time. Because of my success and stability, we're kicking it up a notch! I will be undergoing some additional IV treatments some of them similar to what Lance Armstrong had done during his training. These include an extraction of some of my blood then infusing ozone, nutrients and homeopathies! In addition, I will be getting fitted for structural mouth piece that will assist with appropriately lining up my head, jaw and spinal column. It appears I have some structural issues that may be contributing to my symptoms. And lastly, I will be receiving some structural and visceral manipulation. I'll keep you all posted with more details when I get there.

In the meantime, we are plugging away at getting things done at the house inside and outside. Thanks Dad for hanging pictures and shelves, thanks Julie Izzard for cleaning, Cheryl Hooley for cooking and chopping and dicing foods for my special diet! Thank you, Sue Blankenhagen and Kathy Coveyou for dinners… and Kathy I treasure the therapy pillow covers you and Lillian made me! Hugs to you all. Have a peaceful spring!!! I'm so glad to have a break from that cold white stuff!!!

Living Life to the Fullest
Journal entry by MaryFran Kolp — 6/7/2015

I'm not sure what to write? This has been a full week for certain. Danny finished his last full week of school. He'll be done with his freshman year after finals this week! This weekend he participated in a basketball camp that was held in Kalamazoo and was invitational only, therefore, 80 of the top players in the Midwest were brought together to drill and play hoops. What an experience and honor! If we can keep Danny healthy I see a potential Division one player in our future! Simultaneously, Megan and her AAU basketball team had a tournament in Mt. Pleasant! We have been racking up the miles getting our teens where they need to be!

Through all this Andy's been working and fishing! We had a great walleye dinner last week with family! What a treat!

As for me, I'm preparing to jet set out to California for round two of treatments on Thursday! Prior to my trip, I have appointments, including another MRI scheduled here! I'm trying to stay pumped up, but my left arm weakness has progressed. Again, one day at a time and accept help is all I can do! Here's a funny, my poor husband for the first time ever had to assist me in getting my bra ON when getting dressed! Ha-ha! I needed assistance getting untwisted! We laughed, well kinda. Nevertheless, life goes on! Prayers still forwarded to Darby Walker, Carl

Vanderwall, Lisa Terry, Fred Heiler and their families and all my ALS friends! Love you all!

Back again in Mill Valley, California

Journal entry by MaryFran Kolp — 6/12/2015

We arrived yesterday in San Francisco! Thank you to my escorts Margaret, Jacob and Genevieve Kromm! They have spoiled me! Along with Margaret's brother Andy and his wife Amy Kronk! What a great family! This morning Margaret went to my first doctor appointment with me! I had structural manipulation and visceral adjustments. Dr. Linn utilized visceral, skeletal, and muscular manipulation. Before my appointment I could not raise my left arm up to shoulder level, my neck particularly cervical vertebrae 1,2 and C5 and 6 were all torqued and twisted. Also, I had left ear echoing and left shoulder pain due to atrophy and pinched nerves. After my session with Dr. Linn all of these issues have disappeared or decreased. For the most part just the left arm weakness remains, otherwise all is good! I'm expecting a lot out of this trip, but I too know patience is a virtue! After my appointment, we made a quick stop to Sausalito, had lunch by the water and a cappuccino and organic chocolate! Now I'm back at the hotel resting up! Have a great weekend y'all! Remember "Everybody's got something" so be nice to all you encounter! You are loved unconditionally! How blessed we all are!

Round 2 journey begins

Journal entry by MaryFran Kolp — 6/15/2015

This past weekend I wrote a big part of the last chapter of the book on my divine journey with ALS...I was in the Mill Valley area alone to rest and reflect before treatments began this upcoming week. I look forward to sharing my story and hope that if it provides but even "one positive thing" to future recipients and their caregivers given this diagnosis ...I pray it helps. I thoroughly enjoy and trust my physician team and their staff while on this journey. They not for a moment thought I couldn't beat this or at least feel better and offered support in doing so. Although, like many of you have questioned "Can't you get the same treatments closer to home?" My answer, not before, but maybe now, although it won't be the same. The network of physicians in holistic health and dentistry is really good and the number of patients they treat...amazing! As previously mentioned I have ALS an acronym for many things... A lot of shit, a lot of symptoms, a lot of sickness, amyotrophic lateral sclerosis and the list could go on. Through this process of "unpeeling the onion" removing or correcting symptom by symptom, it appears after 11 months I have not progressed as typical people with ALS progress. Maybe these physicians are on to something in my case. I can't speak for all ALS cases, but mine I can. Why does it appear I'm having success and halt progression? Is it my will to do what God sets in front of me? Is it my ketogenic diet (no grains in 11 months, none) Is it my physician support (thank you for your continued prayers to guide them)? Is it my family and my Frantabulous Friends? Is it the supplements and tinctures and nutritional IV's I'm taking? Is it simply the prayers of those near and far being answered? It could be a combination of the above list. I attribute it to that and that I adopted alternative means of medical treatment. See...when I was first diagnosed in the traditional medical arena, I was told I have ALS. I went for a second opinion, my second opinion agreed with the first and confirmed I had ALS. Then it was recommended I be put on a medication that may possibly extend my life by 2 to 3 months while simultaneously destroying my liver. In addition, I was nicely referred to a support group for my disease. It appeared I was not severe enough to be part of any study at this institution. That was it. Really, no cause, no cure, good luck? This is how I felt with our traditional medical system. I pray this isn't the case with all diagnosed with ALS, but my two friends, I met after my diagnosis: Tammy and Amy with ALS had similar feelings! I would not, nor could I, settle for this outcome. Therefore, I went for a 3rd opinion. I went out of state to a very well-known neurologist who was willing to take a chance and step outside of the box and look at small studies with other patients that had ALS and we created our own protocol. I followed the Deanna protocol with a few extra twists. There it was I was in a study, 1 subject and time would tell! Well, I'm still walking, haven't missed a beat with my kids and their athletic events and traveling, gained 4 lbs, (not characteristic of typical ALS patients), follow my gut with treatments with common sense and try not to dwell on the weakness of my left arm! Focus on the glass half full, not half empty. As for next steps in my treatment plan…this morning I once again had a Bio resonance Analysis of Health assessment. This test by using a blood sample can provide direction for treatment based on the findings. This BAH assessment assists the practitioner in establishing a treatment plan specifically for each patient. In my case, we found I am ready to tolerate more aggressive treatments, IV fusion with ozone. I will receive 2 treatments this week. In addition, I will receive detox IV's on alternate days. I will continue structural treatments and adjustments along with visceral manipulation, lastly, I also received ozone shots and homeopathies in my left jaw today located where my wisdom teeth used to be. A busy week ahead to say the least. It's been great seeing everyone. I've once again been given hope but am ready for a long journey! I'm so grateful for my dear friend and assistant on the remainder of this trip Robin Corrington! Thanks for coming out to be with me! I'll keep you all posted! Thanks for reading! Sorry this was a long one!

Completing my week of treatments in Mill Valley

Journal entry by MaryFran Kolp — 6/17/2015

I want to thank all of you for your positive comments and inspirational thoughts I've received on my CaringBridge site, and text
messages and emails. Don't ever under estimate the power of
prayer and good intentions! They have carried me and my family.
I do apologize for some of my posts being so long winded! I just
have so much to share! I concluded my second visit to Mill Valley
and have completed my physician's recommended treatments
and dental treatments. It has been a long but productive week!
I'm looking forward to starting back home with updated supplements, IVs and most importantly being with my family! This
experience was very interesting, because all of my symptoms
have shown some improvement. I do still have some symptoms
that exist and hope to continue to work on them. This visit I was
stronger, so we took a slightly more aggressive approach in
treatments. As for symptoms that improved or stabilized…feeling
returned to my tongue, improved articulate speech, more energy,
no neck pain, minimized shoulder pain, walking gait more solid,
left arm weakness better but not gone, muscle fasciculations are
predominately in my left side not throughout my body as before.
During this visit I had some unique treatments. I have posted a
few photos in this CaringBridge photo section if you are interested! I too will share the names of these treatments if you are
interested in learning more you can go online to do so. I also
have to share three quick things before considering any judgement on these treatments. 1.) My disease has no cause and no
cure in traditional medicine. 2.) I believe our bodies have limitless
potential if given the right support, to cure, heal, or support itself
within reason…but nothing is impossible. 3.) Consider my results
thus far…I'm not getting worse, possibly better…my treatment
may have implications for those in the future diagnosed with the

symptoms ALS patients typically have, especially in the early stages. The treatments and testing this visit included: ozone injections, autohemotherapy, detoxification IV's, Heavy metals assessment (New finding with testing…some toxic levels of heavy metals and environmental toxins were discovered) structural adjustments, a Bioenergy and resonance assessment to assist in determining my supplemental needs and support specifically. The treatments I feel have had the greatest impact for me were instant relief from ozone injections in the cavitations in my teeth. Within 30 seconds, my ear would crackle and clear after receiving the injection. No doubt one of my many symptoms has a bacterial component and the bacteria is not a good thing for my system in my present state. Another big part of my treatment plan included detoxification IV's and ozone therapies as well. These "cocktails" provided grounding, I didn't feel as uneasy or jittery in my muscular and nervous systems. An interesting result of autohemotherapy or oxygen-ozone therapy (OOT) is when bacteria and viruses die off and toxins released. Typically, minor symptoms similar to the flu, without the fever, can result. So, I did feel a little ill after this treatment. However, in the morning I felt much better. Lance Armstrong must have too after riding the way he did in the tours! The IV ozone infusion I received was similar to Lance's cocktail he was busted for! This journey I was blessed with Margaret Kromm, Jacob and Genevieve escorting me to California and then Robin Corrington flew out to be with me and assist me home! I am so grateful! What blessings you are to me! Back home hugs to my kids and Andy! Special thanks to my in-laws for their help and Sue Blankenhagan for dinner for my family, and Cheryl Hooley for having ketogenic treats ready for me at home upon my return!

Lance Armstrong cocktail
Journal entry by MaryFran Kolp — 6/20/2015

Ozone infusion into my blood with a little saline solution and heparin to prevent blood clotting!

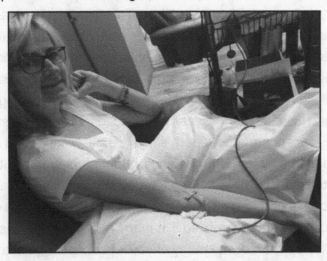

God's promise
Journal entry by MaryFran Kolp — 6/20/2015

"God didn't promise a life without pain, struggles, and hardships. He promises to give you the strength to get through them! "(Faith Reel, twitter) Andy shared this with me tonight! Some of you may need this reflection too! Enjoy!

Happy 4th of July
Journal entry by MaryFran Kolp — 7/3/2015

This week brings back many memories of the past year! First and foremost, I was diagnosed a year ago on my birthday with ALS. What a gift. Ugh, but if I was to receive such terrible information there wasn't a better day to get it as I was surrounded by my family and friends and I only had to share the news once and I didn't have to make numerous calls to those that did not yet know. So, you see it was a blessing. I asked my family and friends to please keep things low key this year for my birthday. Thank you for respecting my wishes. This year has been a lot to process, I can't deny. My birthday has always been a great time my entire life, parties, picnics, presents, fireworks and of course pies and cake! Not to mention family and friends were always around! I love birthdays! This year it was nice to keep things small and intimate, as this year was loaded to say the least! After a year I'm proud to report, since I've been supported more than I deserve by family and friends...through prayer, positive thoughts, financial support for alternative therapies, supplements, hands on support and assistance with our new house and our teens...I have not progressed like many ALS patients. This is a gift. As I've shared with many of you...I will never be able to pay back or pay forward all of the out-of-this-world kindness my family and I have received since my diagnosis. I will not deny, those of you in "my tribe" have seen plenty of tears from me this year! I've tried to adopt Jimmy V's philosophy in his last stages of cancer. He said there are 3 things you should do every day, "first laugh. Laugh every day. Second, think...spend some time in thought daily and third, have your emotions move you to tears!" Works for me! I wanted to share with each of you a gift ...some interesting reading possibly for you or a family member... I've first been inspired by Robin Roberts in her book "Everybody's Got Something". I am keeping all of my journaling and medical notes in hopes I have something to offer those that will encounter neuromuscular conditions in the future. Maybe a book of my own? Second, we have truly decluttered and simplified our stuff, with 3 moves and 2 houses... I enjoyed the book "The Life-Changing Magic of Tidying Up: The Japanese Art of Decluttering and Organizing". And lastly any family with dementia issues, Alzheimer's, MS, ALS or Parkinson's should consider, my now retired from clinical practice Neurologist, Dr. David Perlmutter's publications: "Power Up Your Brain The Neuroscience of Enlightenment." Also, the "Grain Brain" and lastly, his newest publication, just out, "Brain Maker." I believe many answers lie in these observations to our overall health, especially neuromuscular health in the future!

I pray you and your loved ones had a wonderful 4th of July! What a precious celebration for each of us and our country.

Dr. Fran explains some supplements she's taking
Journal entry by MaryFran Kolp — 7/9/2015

Warning! For some of you this entry may be very boring, others intriguing. Supplements 101... Many of you have asked what supplements am I taking and why? This may be boring for many of you, but I've been asked so I'll do my best to share. Because I am an exercise physiologist, with a doctorate in the field, I thought I would attempt explaining what I am taking and why. I will just do a few supplements at a time as to not overwhelm or become too long winded on any one supplement. From my study of the energy production cycles years ago, glycolysis, gluconeogenesis, fatty acid oxidation and others...I understand (or once did) the intermediates in these metabolic cycles and the enzymes that support them. Knowing I was given, a no cause and no cure...therefore no treatment disease, we have opted to provide supplemental support for the intermediates in metabolism in hopes of halting, reversing or slowing the progression of this disease. We know nerves die, muscles go limp, structural support is lost and the end process of physical life is severely shortened. But, if we "unpeel the onion" if you will, and address each potential factor contributing or sustaining this disease...

we may get some control of it. We may not, but it's worth a shot! First, before discussing any supplements, understand I'm on a ketogenic diet. I call it "Atkins diet on steroids". I consume all organics, free range, grass fed stuff I can get my hands on! Including veggies, many meats and fish, tons of nuts, and a lot of healthy fats. Sugars are neurotoxic. Therefore, no sugar, no grains and 1/2 piece of fruit per day. Actually, it's not that hard for me. And as others will agree my skin and my waistline really look good! This ketogenic diet most importantly is neuroprotective! Quickly, a good example of nerve damage from sugars are those most commonly seen in diabetic patients. They lose sensation in limbs and sometimes blindness and amputation can result if sugar levels are not controlled.

The first supplement I am on is developed by Dr. David Perlmutter the author of the" Grain Brain" and other books, and he is also a board-certified Neurologist. This supplement is called nrf2 activator. Nrf2 is a protein messenger carried in every cell of our body. Nrf2 activators presence is necessary to release enzymes necessary to reduce oxidative stress which can be damaging to cells. These enzymes then protect your oligodendrocytes (myelin forming cells) and keep them from dying when under oxidative stress. Anyone with ALS or MS, in my opinion, should be on this support. Google the supplement first and consult with your physician on this before you consider taking it. You may have to educate your physician on this one! Second supplement I take is Inosine. Inosine is a chemical compound found in our bodies. No supplementation is typically required. This compound's main function is to support transfer ribonucleic acid (t-RNA) which supplies polypeptide chains with amino acids. There is some mention Inosine may help nerve branches (axons) grow from healthy nerve cells to injured nerve cells in the brain and the spine. Inosine assists in supporting muscle movement as well, and in some instances is used by body builders. More research is needed on this topic. There can be some side effects even with supplements so again, Google search this and share your findings with your physician prior to taking this. Third to discuss, L-serine powder and Trehalouse. Serine is found in the proteins that make up the brain and it is found in the protective myelinated sheaths that cover our nerves. It is necessary for proper function of our central nervous system and our brain. Deficit serine levels can cause thinning or deterioration of our myelin sheaths that protect our nerves and affects cell communication within the body. Some folks with fibromyalgia and chronic fatigue syndrome have also been noted as having low L-serine levels. Lord knows naps are a huge part of my disorder and adrenal support and serine really helps me...this supplement is my "cup of coffee" midafternoon! Trehalouse is an unusual disaccharide. It's composed of 2 sugars (glucose molecules), it has an unusual bond that can tolerate high temperatures and highly acidic conditions without reducing down in form and also acts as an antioxidant. Lastly for tonight, I can't leave you without one more supplement for the night...adrenal DMG. After extensive blood work on numerous occasions, urine tests, fecal tests and saliva testing. Adrenal burnout was another "layer to my onion". My adrenal glands were in overdrive! Therefore, instead of an "extra shot of expresso" I take Adrenal DMG! Adrenal DMG supports appropriate adrenal function and cortisol levels. Low cortisol symptoms include difficulty getting out of bed in the morning, lack of concentration, anxiety and depression with a twist of indecisiveness! This supplement has been a notable saving grace for me! Speaking of not being able to get up in the morning I best get to bed! We picked up Megan from volleyball camp at U of M and then we're off to Grand Rapids for the first summer league AAU tournament at "Brawl for the Ball"! I'll continue my list tomorrow! Thanks for your continued prayers and support! Sweet dreams!

More supplements... Not kidding!
Journal entry by MaryFran Kolp — 7/10/2015

First and most importantly... Megan had a very successful experience at volleyball camp at U of M! She enjoyed spending time with her cousin Sydney and her childhood -sister- from-another-mother Kira! Ha-ha!! Also, more success for the parallel 45 team Danny is part of in Grand Rapids! They won the first 2 games! Way to go boys! More basketball at 11:30 am tomorrow! Pray they stay healthy and keep winning!

Now onto some more supplements, Glutathione IV, vitamin B12 shot daily, vitamin D. Glutathione naturally occurs in our bodies. It supports our defense system (immune system) in fighting metal and drug poisoning. It is an antioxidant and assists in detoxifying the liver from heavy metal poisoning. I take an oral supplement daily and weekly I also receive a glutathione IV, Andy gives to me. Often after the IV I feel a little flush and light headed. This feeling goes away about 5 to 10 minutes after the IV is administered. I have had some testing done that has revealed I have heavy metals in my system. We're not sure why, some thoughts, Mercury from my amalgam fillings? From immunizations? Environmental toxins... The list goes on! Next, daily I give myself a vitamin B12 shot. At first, I would hunt down anyone that would give me the shot! Now I've graduated and poke myself. Vitamin B12 is a water-soluble vitamin that keeps your nerves and blood cells healthy. If a vitamin B12 deficiency is left untreated it can lead to anemia, causing one to be fatigued and this deficiency can lead to brain damage. I was severely deficit in vitamin B12 and Vitamin D. Vitamin D is made by the body when exposed to sunlight. Also, consumption of vitamin D helps the immune system fight infection, assist with muscle function, cardiovascular and respiratory efficiency functioning and brain development and anti-cancer effects. In a nut shell, vitamin D manages calcium in your gut, blood and bones to ensure your cells communicate efficiently. Time for bed! Have a peace filled night! I'll add some more supplements tomorrow! I'm sure each of you are waiting with bated breath for more...ha-ha! Hugs and good wishes to all.

Supplements continued...
Journal entry by MaryFran Kolp — 7/11/2015

P45 basketball boys are successful again! Won their 11:30 game by 20! Unfortunately, the winning streak ended there! Lost our next game. We made a good effort! Off to Romulus next week-end for more hoops!

On to my list of supplements continued and I'm almost done. Ugh! Ubiquniol CoQ10, Magnesium Taurate, Magnesium Citrate, and Gaba. Ubiquinol CoQ10 is essential in the production of cellular energy. Recall I'm on a ketogenic diet this means my mitochondria (power houses that produce cellular energy) are in overdrive. When CoQ10 is oxidized, it is then used by the body in its reduced form called Ubiquinol. This is the reduced form I choose to take, although our bodies are brilliant and can break-down CoQ10 for cellular use typically, I am taking a reduced form in hopes that my system doesn't have to take that "extra step" to metabolize CoQ10, speculating I'm assisting my system. CoQ10 again exists in a reduced form in our bodies naturally, especially in the heart and liver, muscles and kidneys. Next, magnesium taurate is a scientifically designed amino acid mineral complex to ensure maximal bioavailability of magnesium to my system. I often get muscle cramps when my cell salts are out of balance. Magnesium helps me with this problem. Also, I take magnesium citrate, with all the meat and fiber I consume it ensures regularity! In fact, if you travel and have a tough time going (ha-ha), take some magnesium! It's water soluble so don't be too concerned about overdosing, but be smart, follow the bottle or consult your doctor or the internet for dosing! This should not be used on a regular basis but a little mag citrate on vacation may get you going. GABA is a neurotransmitter that blocks nerve impulses in the brain. This can help to reduce anxiety and may boost mood and have a relaxing effect! Given my diagnosis, regardless of my faith, some stressful moments still occur! I can't deny I'm slowing down a bit! Maybe God's just forcing me to stop and smell the roses along my journey. I hope this Sunday is peace filled for you and your family! Hugs and blessings sent your way! P.S your comments on these posts keep me going! Thank you! I too enjoy hearing back from you!

More supplements & weekend update
Journal entry by MaryFran Kolp — 7/19/2015

We had a great weekend with family! We were downstate for yet another basketball tournament for the parallel 45 team Danny is part of! We stayed at my sister and bro-in-laws (Natalie & Josh's) home in Northville! Then Nat and Josh, Ethan my nephew, Uncle Joel and both Grandparents joined us in cheering on the boys! The team did well. Won one and lost one, this put them in the silver bracket! Then the boys won 2 games and lost in the finals in that bracket! Great job boys! It was a great tournament! A lot of college coaches watching predominantly the upper-class courts. Coach Beilein, Coach Izzo, others from Kent State, Toledo, Oakland, just to name a few. It was pretty cool. Some great ball and players! Off to Indiana this Wednesday! Another big tournament and recruiting mecca!

I also had some hyperbaric treatments this weekend. 3 treatments in two days. This is a process where oxygen is infused into all of your cells, tissues and organs. I watch movies while in the glass encased chamber for 90 minutes. After a treatment once

again, I was whipped, but simultaneously I felt better. My symptoms become more isolated. More under control. My speech is
quicker, my muscle twitching subsides, weakness is still there but
not as extreme. I definitely feel the benefits from hyperbaric treatments. The brain responds favorably to hyperbaric treatment.
Benefits have been documented in patients with Parkinson's,
strokes, brain injuries, and other brain disorders. Recall hyperbaric oxygen therapy empowers mitochondria (power houses
of our cells) to energize the brain. On to supplements... If you
haven't raised your eye brows yet on any of the treatments yet
this may be the first. I have taken some biological (spagyric)
preparations. Spagyric medicine is an advanced form of natural
medication from Europe. Those that I have taken, Cerebretik
(brain support), Hepatik (liver support), Lymphotik (lymphatic
support) and Renalin (kidney support). Many medications act
to relieve and manage symptoms. The "Soluna" medicines act
in a deep systematic way, regulating proper functioning on a
cellular level in restoring health by homeopathy, herbology and
pharmacology. Each medicine targets a specific system or organ
to assist in restoring proper function so that disease no longer
persists, and symptoms naturally stop. Each of these medicines
from Germany combines numerous high-quality plants, herbs,
minerals, and metallic elements, and undergo a scientific process to produce a highly concentrated and bioavailable product.
These liquid tinctures were taken twice a day for 30 days. Some
taste OK, others downright nasty! Nevertheless, I haven't progressed like typical ALS patients. Maybe there are some things
that folks can do to help and support themselves when given
such an extreme diagnosis? Encourage those you meet that are
given the "I don't know what to tell you" line from a physician...
To find another opinion/ physician, try alternative care (check
certification and backgrounds) there may be some answers for
you after all... And a lot more questions! (Ha-ha) Good luck!

Extras above supplements
Journal entry by MaryFran Kolp — 7/21/2015

This past weekend we went to Indiana for an AAU basketball
tournament with Danny! What a season these boys from the
north have had! If you are a basketball fan in general, Fort
Wayne, Indiana is a basketball mecca! In this national championship tournament Danny's division 15U for the tournament had 44
teams! Basketball everywhere! At this tournament we had a few
dreams come true for our son this weekend... Not that anything
will come of it but it gives us and him hope for the future, as for
what this was...Tom Izzo, the head coach from MSU came to
watch Danny play. We were given the heads up he may do this...
He couldn't believe it, nor could we, looking up in the coaching
and recruiting stands and there he was! Danny and the team
played well too and won! Way to go boys from the north. That
wasn't all, in addition to that highlight, Bacari Alexander from U
of M watched another game of Danny's at the Spiece Center and
stayed for the entire game. To top that off, Oakland University's,
recruiting coach Drew Valentine watched 3 of Danny's games.
Also, Northwestern, Central Michigan University and University
of Detroit recruiters were in the stands! It's nice to know Danny's
being recognized. Being "on the radar" at this point is a gift!
A special thank you to Danny's coach and Sports journalist,
Steve Bell for getting him on the "who to watch for the future"
list. As Danny grows and gets stronger...the sky's the limit for
him! Time will tell! Now switching gears here's the final listing of
my supplements: Brain sustain, ProDHA, DHEA and A-L complex immune support. First, Xymogen BrainSustain, developed
by Dr. Perlmutter to support brain health. It's a vanilla shake
that provides support for the brain and spine. proDHA provides
neurological support and brain support. DHEA in my case may
help with my adrenal insufficiency, as my adrenal glands are

exhausted! Can you blame them? I saw another very well-known physician in Ann Arbor, Dr. Neuenschwander utilizing holistic health practices. It will be nice to have someone that supports alternative therapies for neuromuscular disorders closer to home. I was put on a cancellation list and was blessed with a call and by divine intervention we met today! I will undergo further testing, but it appears there are many factors contributing to my ALS symptoms, such as, bacteria such as those associated with Lyme disease, heavy metals such as mercury and a compromised immune system. Further testing will offer next steps for my treatment. I am still down state and will be for the next week. In addition, I will be getting hyperbaric treatments and starting at home detox IV's and Danny will be attending two invitational basketball camps! Lansing and Detroit here we come! Hugs to all of you reading!

Just a friendly update
Journal entry by MaryFran Kolp — 7/31/2015

While Danny is attending a day camp in Lansing, I took this perfect opportunity to visit Darby Walker, a young lady Danny's age from Petoskey with cancer. She is presently at Sparrow Hospital undergoing chemotherapy. I was blessed to go to lunch with Shawn, her Mom. Darby had a spinal today and with prayers they were successful with one poke! Darby is a strong little lady, I get strength and hope from her and watching her journey, while living mine! Just thought I'd put it out there, if you have an extra prayer or two, we'll take them! We are so blessed... And we've experienced firsthand prayers help!!! Remember everybody's got something! Celebrate today! Have a Margarita for us (I can do organic tequila and limes... Ha-ha)! Or a lemonade if you prefer!!! Thank you for your kind comments on my CaringBridge site! They continue to inspire me!

Back home with family and friends
Journal entry by MaryFran Kolp — 8/2/2015

Today was a wonderful gift! After celebrating Mass at the parish
I grew up in, I was able to see and receive many heartfelt hugs
and blessings from neighbors and friends I grew up with! I kind of
revert back to a kid seeing all of them and this group of neighbors
or "adopted family members by my heart" felt a peacefulness
being amongst these precious people that know my history, my
strengths and weaknesses and still find it in their hearts to pray
for me and my family! I can never thank them enough, except to
offer up prayers for all of them and their loved ones. Which I will
do! Danny and my parents and I went to breakfast with this group,
once referred to as "The South Lyon Yacht Club Members" and
had an enjoyable meal! It has been a long while since I've seen
many of them! It was good to catch up if even for a brief time. The
fun didn't end there, I had a wonderful afternoon with childhood
friends and their families! Danny and I went to the Burke's home
(Pam Heiler Burke) one of my ultimate best friends growing up
and the Skene family came over too! (Tracy Meloche-Skene) my
best granola friend, wise beyond her years and our kids have
grown up during summers together! It was a great afternoon! And
Doug, Danny has you by at least 2 inches! Lol. Alright…you have
him by at least 149 lbs!!! Today was a blessing! I am grateful!
What a special day! All Sunday afternoons should be spent simi-
larly! I pray all of you reading had a great weekend!

Hyperbaric and treatment update
Journal entry by MaryFran Kolp — 8/5/2015

This week I have been doing double sessions in the hyperbaric
oxygen chambers in South Lyon, my home town. Living back
home getting spoiled by Mom and Dad! While Danny lived at my

sister's! She has Wi-Fi and Uncle Josh too is there, along with the cousins! Honestly, this week started out rough, I didn't feel really strong and I was very tired. Between Dr. appointments, hyperbaric, seeing friends and family along with getting Danny to basketball camp in Dearborn (thanks dad & mom and Carl for help driving him)!

I did have the honor of meeting with Dr. Neuenschwander "Dr. Neu" he's a very kind physician that works with patients with neurological disorders and those with Lyme disease in Ann Arbor. He is located at the Bio Energy Medical Center. We are re-running my Igenx Western Blot Lyme's panel. As last year there were some insignificant bands indicating its possible presence. But, nothing positive according to CDC guidelines. I'm curious of this result now as Lyme disease may be contributing to my disease symptoms. This does not mean if I have Lyme disease that my ALS diagnosis will go away, but some of my symptoms may be treatable. In addition, Dr. Neu ordered more blood work and a urine sample to assess some other things in my blood and potential heavy metals in my system. While doing this I also received double sessions of hyperbaric treatments as already mentioned. These treatments exhaust me, but also, they make me feel like my symptoms are more refined, specifically to my left arm and shoulder. My legs are weak but after a little rest, I feel so much better!

As for Danny's camp…it was a great experience. He had drills in small groups and attended lectures regarding, character and integrity, setting a high standard for yourself, recruiting, sports nutrition, importance of academics in high school and college, offenses, choices in personal relationships, they covered the spectrum of topics! They also had a career day and went to the Lion's training facility and met some players. In addition, they went to Quicken loans to get an education on financial information and how to be careful with finances. Danny also had great conversation with coaches and professional players, Tim McCormick

(Randy, Eric and Dan…Danny told Tim hello for you, he sends his best to you guys) also, Lindsey Hunter! This camp was an honor and privilege for Danny! He made great contacts and played with some of the top 100 high school kids in the state! Danny even moved up and played with the Michigan elite 17 and 18 year-old's! These boys sure were big! Danny looked average sized compared to them but played very well! Danny and I head home tomorrow!

Journal entry by MaryFran Kolp — 8/20/2015

Will Edison has an interesting piece on You Tube.

"Rise to Greatness: Fearless Faith." Watch it. If you have something you're working through or something troubling you, hopefully this will be a message to help you on your journey. It was good for me to watch today.

I don't have any blood test or other test results back yet. I was told 4 to 6 weeks, so I will call next week and hopefully have some answers then. What I have been doing are continued supplements, detox IV's at home (prescribed by my physicians in California), and acupuncture. Also visiting the eye doctor thanks Tess and Sarah from Infinity Eye Care, my prescription with hyperbaric treatment changes drastically for about 3 weeks and they have multiple lenses on site for me! Besides a few bumps in the road, honestly, it's been a fantastically blessed summer, but a challenging few weeks. Andy had to assist me in pulling up some tight shorts, getting my sweatshirt on and shaving my arm pits this week! Ugh! My left arm is I could say "really weak" or "maximally being put on detox duty to try and keep me as well as God permits." Included in this detox process I have cried A LOT. All kinds of tears, happy, sad, blessed, fearful and just feeling like PMS on steroids in the crying arena!

Every night I count my blessings and try to reflect on what gifts I was given that day! But, I am human and must admit "fear of what the future holds for me and my kids and my beloved

husband of 19 years crept in the past few weeks." We just celebrated our Anniversary! I'm so blessed Andy meant it when he
said he'd love me in sickness and health. This anniversary was
different, no golf or biking this year…we went to Mission Peninsula
and Traverse City! We walked, wine tasted, had a great dinner
at the Jolly Pumpkin and talked about our wedding and sharing
that day with those we love! I do freak-out from time to time but
not in front of my kids. What gets me through are YOUR prayers,
YOUR gifts from God shared with my family and me. For example,
I received a very thoughtful card and have received others from
Norm and Emily Daniels. They pray for me and I guess God gets
a pen in Emily's hand and when I'm full of more fear than faith
she writes, and I get a card in perfect timing for my need. They
are St. Francis Parish family members that have adopted us in
prayer and we have adopted them in family! I am so blessed to
have them and all of you! We have had spectacular meals, Sue
Blankenhagen my family loves your meatloaf and the mashed
potatoes! Marie Law thanks for keeping me on track with appointments and starting to organize more of our stuff! Melody Collins
and Terri Reynolds, Annette Pocica and team Maggie Kromm
and Trudy Haussman Hogan, thanks for making our house look
like a home! Melody you truly knocked it out of the ballpark. Your
connections and shopping skills to decorate my house is amazing. I'll post a few pictures here too. I've decided to go away more
often! Ha! Every time I go away someone redecorates or does
something spectacular with our house. I call our house the "pizza
house"! All are welcome, and our home is a safe-haven for all
teens living out of town and waiting for a practice or after school
activity! We are in the perfect location across from the high school
and many families and friends from this community helped us put
together this house. The least we can do to give back in thanks
and have an open door! We are so appreciative and grateful!
Hugs to All of you! Remember the glass is always half full!

Danny's playing Varsity Tennis

Journal entry by MaryFran Kolp — 8/22/2015

Great first tournament! Even a picture in the News Review! How blessed!

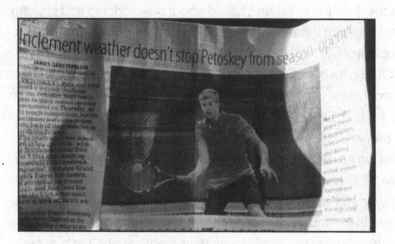

Megan's Freshman volleyball team undefeated champions

Journal entry by MaryFran Kolp — 8/22/2015

Congratulations Northwomen!

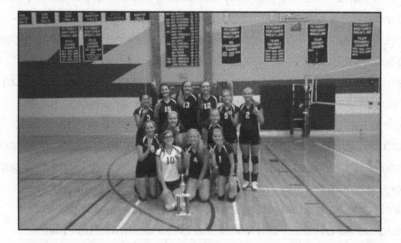

Congratulations Megan!

Journal entry by MaryFran Kolp — 8/22/2015

The Petoskey tournament held this weekend was a great success! Undefeated Petoskey Freshman against Sault St. Marie, Elk Rapids, TC St. Francis, Boyne City! Way to go girls!

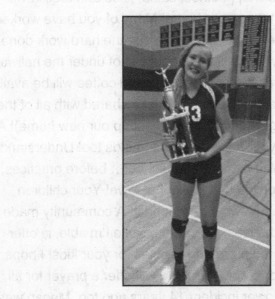

News a Mom has to share

Journal entry by MaryFran Kolp — 8/25/2015

This was a most memorable day! Andy, Danny, and I went to Central Michigan University on an unofficial recruiting visit for basketball today! After a tour of the facilities, meetings with Coach Smith and Coach Davis and Taylor the strength trainer, a tour of the sports complex, dorms, and the business school Danny was given an offer to play basketball there! Go Chips! It was an honor and privilege for Danny! We are so blessed! He has a lot to think about!

Kolp Open House after dropping kids to school!
Journal entry by MaryFran Kolp — 9/1/2015

Mark your calendars the first Friday of school, Sept. 11 join us 8:30-11am at the Kolp's home for a back to school catch-up from the summer time! Quiche, pastries, salad, juice and tequila will be here for breakfast & see our home! Many of you have worked on this house and we thank you! Come see the hard work done by friends and family! We will do a tequila shot under the hallway chandelier promptly at 9am! Other shots and coffee will be available too! (The tequila shot has been a joke shared with all of the hard workers moving us and helping to set up our new home)! All are welcome! Bring your back to school friends too! Understand your children are welcome here after school… before practices, especially for those of you that live out of town! Your children always have a home in town if they need it! A community made this house a home, the least we can do, while I'm able, is offer our home and unlimited pizza and veggies for your kids! I hope to see many of you on Sept. 11th…we will offer a prayer for all involved in the twin tower incident 14 years ago too. Megan was 2 weeks old!

Stem cells a possibility on the horizon
Journal entry by MaryFran Kolp — 9/1/2015

More than 115 million dollars were brought in doing the ALS ice bucket challenge! Many of you contributed to this cause…and I thank you…especially to those challenges personally dedicated to me…nevertheless I think it's CRAZY pouring ice over yourselves! Ha! But what an outcome to this crazy effort! There's a lot of applicable research now out there and I like to think I'm just a small sample to the cutting edge holistic alternative solutions to this problem! Between numerous tests (FDA approved and others not), a ketogenic diet, supplements, acupuncture, cranial sacral therapy, walking daily, homeopathies, detox IV's, dental cavitations addressed, hormone issues, metal detox, support from a physician team who believes the body has a great capacity to heal if given the tools! Now I am preparing to find out more about stem cell injections. I would not receive embryonic stem cells, I would receive an injection of my own stem cells into my spinal areas affected. To find out more on who I will be seeing and a brief description of what I have done to prepare for this I encourage you to Google...strokedoctor.com. Dr. David Steenblock, DO has a stem cell research lab and stem cell therapy protocol for ALS patients in southern California. As you will see in his ALS video, this is a multifaceted disease (kind of like unpeeling the onion as previously described by me). My physicians in California are supportive in finding out more and creating a plan. This will be as expected, expensive. We will keep you all informed on how you may be able to contribute or help down the line. Don't think I've given up and am doing stem cell injections as a last resort. I'm not. This is just another chapter in the book I'm determined to write in hopes it can help others yet to be diagnosed!

September 11th...It's been 14 years...
Journal entry by MaryFran Kolp — 9/10/2015

Seems like yesterday when Megan was born. September 11th happened two weeks after her birth. Is hard to believe it's been over 14 years now since the twin towers fell in New York City. This is just a reminder those of you in town after you drop off your kids to school stop on by, if possible, to have a little breakfast, a little prayer session and a shot of tequila under the chandelier! I look forward to seeing all of you that can join us! Bring a friend! Well Megan has started high school and is thoroughly enjoying it! In addition, she is doing very well with her volleyball team! They defeated Traverse City West last evening in two straight games! Danny also is doing great! He continues to get phone calls from other colleges, Iowa, UC Davis, Vanderbuilt, that are interested in him for basketball! He's doing double sessions working out for tennis and creating a basketball routine for coaches coming to see him as a person and a player. His tennis season in high school is also going very well. Also, he got his license this week! Not many can say they got a scholarship offer before getting their driver's license! Lol. It goes to show you when you work hard and use the gifts God has given you, nothing is impossible! Danny is getting ready to go to a tennis tournament this weekend in Midland and Meg will have a volleyball tournament this weekend as well in Kalkaska! No grass growing under the Kolps' feet! Andy is such a hard worker and trooper. We are so blessed to have him! As for me, just like you, I go day by day. I am planning another trip to California at the end of October where we will be moving forward with IVs and treatments and discussing stem cells. I can't thank you enough for all your love, help and support. All your help we can't even begin to thank you! Just know, if I make it through this it's because of angels like you and the pure grace of God! Hopefully, all our efforts, especially those of you praying will reap the benefits of our works! I hope all of you have had a great kick start to the new school year and I pray you and your family had a fabulous summer!

September 11th recap
Journal entry by MaryFran Kolp — 9/12/2015

It was great to see those of you that made it yesterday! We prayed for and offered a toast under the hall chandelier for the victims and all of the caregivers as promised! 24 Moms and Lillian in total showed! It was so nice to catch up! I think we're going to meet the first Friday of each month and catch up over coffee and juices! The location may change, probably "coffee shop hop" I'd guess month to month! Here's a start… October 2nd North Perk's, November 6, Roast and Toast! Like my husband says sick or not…if I'm not going to a party I'm throwing one! Just join if you can! No pressure! All are welcome! Drop you kids and come for a cuppa Joe!!! Lol. Hugs and blessings to all of you! Have a great weekend! It's a beautiful fall day in Kalkaska!!!

September activity update from the Kolps

Journal entry by MaryFran Kolp — 9/26/2015

This fall, thus far, has been beautiful and amazing! Danny's tennis season has been very successful, and he's enjoyed it! Megan's volleyball team too has been doing very well! We are so blessed by the athletic and academic success by them! In addition, Danny's still on the radar for potential collegiate basketball opportunities. Iowa is coming to see him and meet his coaches this Tuesday. Crazy but in God's hands this recruiting adventure is! As for Andy all is well. He had an unfortunate funeral for his GVSU assistant coach, Bill Springer this past week. He drove to Grand Rapids and had a blessed visit with old players, trainers and coaches. I know for certain many great fun stories, laughs and remembrances were shared! RIP coach, you made a difference in these old boys' lives! We had another special gift this weekend, our niece Dana came home from MSU for the weekend and stayed with us! It was wonderful to catch up! As for my health update, I have restarted my detox IV's. They kick my butt initially but after about 2 days I have more energy and feel better. I am still doing supplements, no pharmacy ALS drugs at this point, by my choice. To date, for me the risks of increased bodily endangerment isn't worth the additional 2 extra months of life from these meds. Just nutrients and metabolic intermediates are what I'm taking. In addition to note, and an interesting point, a few months prior to my diagnosis I had stopped having a menstruation cycle. Thinking I was on my way into menopause, however as of the last 6 months, it has returned, not missing a beat. I only share this, not to gross the male readers out, but to state a fact, with my improved health could this be a positive thing for me? Systems not absolutely, necessary working again. Could continuing to peel the layers of health issues help me and those women in the future with this diagnosis? We don't know. The experts don't know, but I think it's worthy to note. I have appointments up and coming, neurologist mid-October, a biological dentist I found in Michigan that may be able to assist in continuing ozone treatments in my dental cavitations. Many dentists are skeptical about dental cavitations. In my case, skeptical or not, once I receive an ozone shot I have instant relief of my echoing left ear and an instant change in my neck which feels much more relaxed and less tense. This change usually only last for 10 hours but, is that something also that should be noted? Is any relief an indication that there is a possible bacterial variable contributing to my disease. Again, no one knows for sure. In addition, discussion about removing my remaining amalgam fillings will be addressed. Amalgam fillings contain toxins, mercury for one, and heavy metals may too be a contributing factor. Therefore, these will be addressed. Lastly, Andy and I will be doing a quick trip to touch base with my doctors in California at the end of October! I pray all is well for you and your families! Please keep us in your prayers, as you too are in ours! Hugs to all of you!

Journal entry by MaryFran Kolp — 10/11/2015

Things are moving along at the Kolps. Andy and I had a great spontaneous trip to Mackinac Island! Great walking, talking and drinking and eating! We love the island! While my left side becomes progressively weaker, the Kolp kids are cranking, and we're moving forward! God has them in the palm of his hand. This weekend was crazy busy! I unfortunately had to miss my South Lyon High School class reunion and other festivities, as I had a terrible respiratory infection and Andy was work-ing, Megan had a volleyball tournament and Danny had tennis regionals and Iowa came to visit this afternoon to see Danny and meet his coach and his family. In summary, I'm feeling better, not coughing as much. Danny's tennis team won region-als and we'll be going to the state meet next week in Holland! Megan's team won the JV volleyball tournament in Harbor Springs! Lastly, Danny's recruiting visit with Coach Francis from Iowa went well. We will be going to visit Iowa's campus later this fall! For those of you in the downstate area Thursday, November 12th...My sister has arranged a fundraising opportunity for my potential stem cell treatment. John Heffron, a friend who we went to high school with, and is a comedian from LA now, is will-ing to help by donating his proceeds from Royal Oak Comedy Castle. A silent auction and games are also in the making. More details will follow shortly! We are so grateful! God is good!

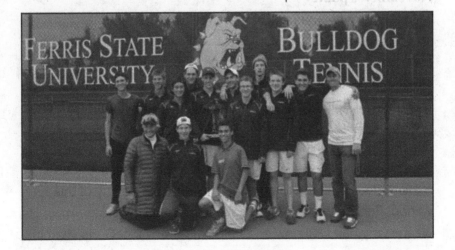

Petoskey volleyball tournament champs!

Journal entry by MaryFran Kolp — 10/11/2015

The Freshman Petoskey volleyball team won the JV tournament in Harbor Springs!

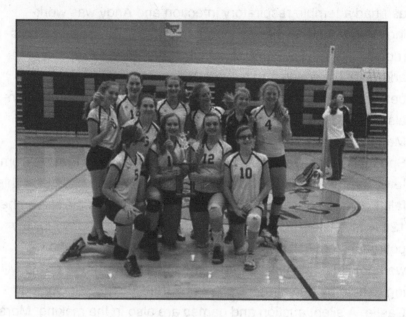

November Update

Journal entry by MaryFran Kolp — 11/2/2015

I learned in direct sales some people choose looking at life situations either on the "light" train or the "dark" train. I choose to ride the light train being positive, living in the moment and being grateful. Others ride the dark train, the cup is half empty, negative thoughts, blaming others for their troubles. Some days I do get sad and feel sorry for myself, I'm human and this has been a tough deck of cards to be dealt! How people do any of this without Faith is beyond me. I have learned a lot, as has Andy! He washes my hair well now and helps me dress too! Sorts vitamins and supplements and makes beds! We had a beautiful wedding, but our marriage has been my greatest treasure! Andy is a great man and caregiver. Think about how hard it must be, being a physician and not being able to fix or cure your ill wife. I feel for him. On a lighter side… I've learned it's easier going without a bra now that we're in layer dressing season, also thong under- wear make it much easier to pull up pants when your arms are challenged, than the typical woman's jockey cotton undies I'm used to! It's been quite a month. I received a confirmed diagnosis of ALS from the Director of the ALS clinic at U of M. I'm progress- ing although not as quick as most. I have been encouraged to keep doing what I'm doing. I suppose that's a good thing. I use my left arm minimally and now feeling some effects in my right arm and my legs at times. Still have some issues to address like metal toxins, cavitations…so time will tell. I had a great trip with my husband to his conference in Florida, followed by a trip back to Mill Valley, California to do follow up appointments with my physicians out there. We were blessed to stay in San Francisco with Maggie Kromm's brother and sister in-law and their family! We are so blessed and they were so kind, welcoming and gra- cious! Thank you, Andrew and Amy! This saved us so much. I received structural adjustments, supplement revisions, detox IV updates, stem cell next steps discussion, ozone treatments and OSB mouth piece adjustments. Now I am home and whipped! I have cavitations surgery and amalgam fillings removal scheduled later this month. I'm so looking forward to and grateful for the upcoming fundraising event and seeing family and friends and John Hefferon, the well-known comedian from LA my sister and I went to school with. He's hilarious! It will be a great fun evening! I hope you and friends will consider coming Thursday, November 12th to Mark Ridley's Comedy Castle, Royal Oak. Doors open at 5:30. Food 6pm. Live auction 7-7:15. John on stage at 8pm!!!

Contact Natalie Reed for tickets. Tickets are not available at the door.

Andy and Danny and Megan are doing well! The kids have had some quality time with my folks and Aunt Terri and Uncle Craig while we've been away! How blessed we all are! The kids finished fall sports. Danny had a great tennis season, the team won Regionals and placed 13th as a team at States. Megan's volleyball team won their league and won 4 of the tournaments they were in this fall! Now hoop season begins mid-November for both kids! Danny's still being recruited by more colleges, Oakland and CMU came to visit while Andy and I were gone. Toledo and Xavier have expressed interest as well. This season will be a big one for Danny! Pray all stay healthy!!! Hugs to each of you thanks for all of your help and support!

Fund-raiser update and laughs

Journal entry by MaryFran Kolp — 11/13/2015

Who remembers Harmony House? Waiting all day to hear a favorite song? When short shorts were in for guys? And lyrics to 1980's music? Not children born of the Millennium Age with I-phones!!! I do believe laughter is the best medicine! And we were blessed with good laughs last night! John Hefferon, a well-known comedian grew up with us in the 1980's in South Lyon and now residing in LA, had a fabulous performance! He had the ability to teach life lessons with humor across the age spectrum! Hilarious!!! A special thank you to John for his generosity and financial support at the fund-raiser last evening. An extra special thank-you to all of you that donated and took the time out for a hug or to say hello last evening. I was even blessed by Andy's twin sister coming into town for the event! While shopping and laughing with my niece Dana and my sisters-in-law that took great care of me Terri, Paula and Elena! Thank you! It's been a while since I've seen many of you and it's such a bummer or should I say blessing I have this disease? It was so good to see all of you that were able to attend the fund-raiser! Many family members came, some folks I grew up with, college friends and some supporters I didn't even know! The support and the love Andy and I felt was indescribable! In part many of the friends and colleagues were there because of our hosts: Josh and Natalie Reed, my generous brother in-law and my loving, driven sister. To know them is to love them! They both work full-time, have great kids that are very busy and care for friends and family and have a beautiful home! Through all this they took on putting on a fund-raiser for me! I know if they could take this challenge away from me they would! I know this has been difficult being so far away. They hosted a great successful event at Mike Ridley's comedy castle, catered food, invited David Santia, from Detroit to do speed painting for entertainment and auction! Had a beautiful silent auction with a variety of items, sealed by a Heffron performance! This was so cool! Also, Natalie bought me my outfit to wear and a friend bought a gift certificate to the spa for hair and make-up (no Andy didn't do my hair and make-up, nor did he dress me for this event-lol)! What was all this for and how did it go? For those curious, it appears my dental costs not covered by insurance will cost approximately $5,000 this includes: cavitation surgery, 6 amalgam filling removals, homeopathies, and hyperbaric treatments! All happening before the end of the year! In addition, stem cells as previously mentioned, the entire procedure and follow-up will cost over $40,000 again no insurance coverage for experimental stem cell research using my stem cells! These treatments were not feasible before this event, and are not for many other ALS patients, Natalie and Josh knew that…with your help and contribution we brought in approximately $25,000 so far!!!!!! As I've mentioned before, "Divine Interventions". God has me on a journey…with my progress and improvement because of treatments you're giving me the opportunity to do; I hope my story and my path of ALS control and possible remission will be used to share with those in the future diagnosed and that have it now! From me and future persons with ALS…Thank you! I will keep you posted on your investment! We love and thank you and will continue to pray for each of you and your families.

Happy Thanksgiving! Blessings & Good Wishes
Journal entry by MaryFran Kolp — 11/25/2015

I sincerely hope you and your families have a spectacular Thanksgiving! As the holidays are upon us please take some time for YOU and cut back on your to do lists! Only make 5 different cookies not 10! Decorations… Simplify! Cards…send to older folks that appreciate them and to those that will keep them! Otherwise, Facebook your Christmas wishes and kid pictures to friends! Visit with family and friends, be present and stop making ourselves crazy!!!! Before I got sick I would NOT have taken to heart my recommendations. I thought I was expected to do it all! I didn't want to disappoint anyone; especially myself…I like to run on adrenalin!!! I hope you will be different, for your health and enjoyment!

I'm so grateful and appreciate all your prayers, kind comments on this blog and financial support for my health expenses. These are some of the things I'm thankful for, as many of you know, we've simplified at the Kolp house, but the medical bills have been a burden. I realize I'm not alone in this concern. Many people struggle with bills. I pray for those struggling especially during the holidays. I have a precious story that pulled on my heartstrings! My brother in-law and sister's friend's son, named Reed, is a young boy with a heart of gold! He remembered Danny and when Reed was told Danny's mom was sick he asked his mom if he could donate his own money to me. His mom allowed it and I am so touched beyond tears! This is one of MANY stories of thanks and gratitude. As I've said before, I have felt more love than I deserve. I pray my whole journey allows me to give back to those suffering. Keep the prayers coming! I thank all of you I know and those I don't know…that still gave and prayed! I'm speechless!

I still think of John Heffron's comedy act often! I'm getting many friends "post it notes and mini Patron tequila" for gifts. So, everyone can write and leave love notes and reminders to loved ones in the new year! Lol. Just like John shared with us in his comedy skit! The Patron is my contribution… Even though there's snow…I love a good Margarita!

I have begun my dental visits in preparation for removing amalgam fillings and cavitation's surgery. Thank you, Maggie Kromm for escorting me downstate! And Robin Corrington for hosting us and driving me to hyperbaric oxygen treatments! I've started them again! Three more weeks of dental prep, hyperbaric treatments and traveling downstate! Then stem cell implementation will be addressed in the new year! Without your support, honestly, I wouldn't have been able to even consider these treatments. I'm beyond thankful! I'll keep you posted! Don't forget to consider simplifying this holiday season…or at least consider it! Happy Thanksgiving! Hugs, love and blessings being sent your way!

Merry Christmas and Happy New Year from The Kolp Family

Journal entry by MaryFran Kolp — 12/19/2015

Have you ever been part of a "pay it forward" experience? Many have heard of this happening but how many have experienced it? My good friend and hostess/caregiver Robin Corrington from downstate and I went to a drive through Starbucks and the person in front of us, who we did not know, nor did we get to thank, paid the bill! We in turn did the same for the lady behind us!!! What a feel-good moment it was! Very kind! Thank you too all the secret Santa givers! I know all of us are in the middle of the hustle and business of the season… But don't forget the true meaning of the season and focus on the people, not the stuff!!! This evening we are having our "Frantabulous Friends" over for cocktails and hors d'oeuvres! I would have truly enjoyed having all of you but were in a smaller home this year. Nevertheless, we are so thankful for all of the support and prayers! This particular group, which many of you are a part, have signed up to facilitate my care needs and our family's needs over the year. Each family has between 3 and 4 weeks a year they have designated to help. We're so grateful for all the help, food, contributions, shopping, supplement sorting, road trips downstate, laundry folding, vacuuming, etc.! It's been surreal! Remember if you have a loved one in need get the "Share the Care" book. It's been an amazing process for us and beyond words helpful, especially that now I'm needing more care! I'm not sure if I'm getting weaker from disease or just freezing up from the snow and cold! God has my back I'm taking one day at a time. Last Monday I did have my amalgam fillings taken out! All 6 of them, 2 were cracked, hopefully with the removal I too will notice a positive effect! Interesting process for me, I had ozone shots and hyperbaric treatments 4 consecutive weeks prior to the removal! When being prepared for the actual removal of my fillings; which include silver, mercury and other toxins, I was draped with a cover, put on a hair net and a mesh screen over my face sealed with an oxygen mask! In addition, the dentist and hygienist had masks on and looked like they were from the planet Mars! Lastly, a vacuum suction hose was placed close to my mouth to ensure any toxic gases or amalgam power would be absorbed. What a process to take precautions. Note I had been told through blood testing and muscle testing that I have heavy metals in my system. With my health issues I didn't mind the precautions taken, but I'm glad it's over! After the new year I will have my wisdom teeth cavitation surgery… Then we'll re-access and discuss next steps with my team of physicians. I pray you and your family are well and really enjoy each other this holiday season! We all are so blessed but often forget all the gifts we have!!! Forgive me! This is my Christmas Card this year! Hugs and blessings from the Kolp family today and throughout the year! …a few pictures of Danny and Megan to follow! God bless us! Merry Christmas and Happy New Year!

Fund-raiser with John Hefferon
Journal entry by MaryFran Kolp — 12/19/2015

Natalie Reed my sister and friends Michele Bird and Julie Nadeau!

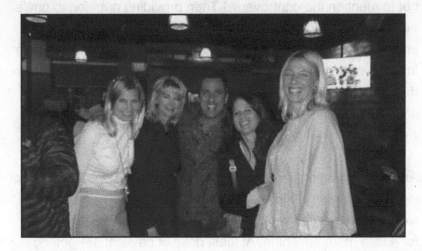

Happy 2016
Journal entry by MaryFran Kolp — 1/4/2016

I hope all of you had a very blessed holiday season! Great
Thanksgiving, Christmas, Hanukkah, Kwanzaa and a Happy New
Year! Remember to graciously put away all the holiday garb!
You're blessed to have it! I was blessed with my Christmas elves
coming over yesterday to tear down our Christmas house. It was
so beautiful! Andy and I were so grateful for the help! Switching
gears... I have cavitation surgery scheduled January 26th. Not
looking forward to that but it needs to be done. I'm hanging in
there! I'm still walking but upper weakness continues to increase.
Andy and friends do much for me these days. Good News! I
have discovered there are now some STEM cell studies being
conducted in the states, Mayo and Massachusetts for starters.
I will be investigating more this week. These STEM studies are
again using one's own STEM cells, not embryonic, there have
been very few if any success stories with embryonic studies,
not to mention the controversy! Then providing nutrition to one's
own stem cells and resubmitting into one's spine. Noticeable
improved functional changes have been noted in a month's time
in some subjects in European studies. Let's hope this is a break-
through!!! I'll keep you posted! Hugs and blessings to all of you!

Journal entry by MaryFran Kolp — 1/21/2016

Anyone wondering if we have snow up north? Absolutely!!! Great
skiing for Northern Michigan! Many are enjoying the "powder"
we've been blessed with! Nevertheless, I've put my order in
for a little more sunshine! At least days of daylight are getting
longer! As for updates...I once again thank all of you for your
prayers, donations and support! I am so far behind on thank-
you notes, forgive me! With the help of friends Deanna, Kim and

Janet, I have forwarded to those that wrote checks for me a brief thank-you for the comedy fund-raiser. We were so touched and grateful. What an awesome event it was! We too are hoping for a "Hail Mary" when it comes to this ALS stuff! Your contribution is helping in this goal! Mrs. Elliot and the prayer group at the Methodist Church, I thank you and treasure the prayer blanket given to me. It is beautiful, and you were very kind to pray for me. As for medical updates, I had my blood work drawn for preliminary evaluation at the request of the STEM cell treatment center in California. They extracted 11 vials of blood! Results are now in and forwarded to my respective physicians. I'll find out more next week. I still have a few other tests to do but with all of the other treatments involving my dental cavitations, I'm not ready to go off supplements for 3 days at this point. Which is what I need to do prior to any additional testing asked of me. In the meantime, I had intense ozone treatments in preparation for my cavitation surgery next week. The biological dentist I've been working with is excellent and I have a great respect for him. My treatment this time included shots in my mouth 2-3 on the left and right where my wisdom teeth used to be. Then 4 shots on the left and right exteriorly where my lymph nodes are located. By and behind my left ear where all my symptoms started. Then lastly my left shoulder and scapular area where atrophy has really set in. This all was then followed by a nasal/auricle treatment of ozone as well. Ozone has a distinct scent and flavor. Not good nor bad, but I've had enough to recognize it. This cleansing and detoxifying agent I respond well to. My ear crackling or echoing stops right away and although still weak my disease feels more refined in my arms and shoulders. Time will tell with these treatments and detoxification homeopathies I've been put on. Next week I will have cavitation surgery and more ozone treatments along with hyperbaric oxygen treatments as well.

Our kids are doing well! Megan had a team building

sleepover in Saginaw this weekend and a defense volleyball clinic and a hitting specialty clinic in Midland with her team. Danny will be back on the court this week after struggling with a pinched nerve in his back. Thanks Rob, Shelly, Christy and Grant of Orthosport for assisting Danny in the healing process! I want to thank all my Frantabulous Friends and angels here for me and my family. The meals, support, prayers, communion, rides, driving, cleaning, folding, hair help, dressing me, preparing my food, shopping and laughing with me and crying with me…thank you! P.S. my tears are in part for what I'm losing and what's slipping away, but most of my tears are just in complete thanks and awe that I'm so blessed to have all the help and support I do! You each are a divine intervention for me!

Cavitation surgery is over!
Journal entry by MaryFran Kolp — 1/28/2016

I want to first thank all of you that have posted comments on this blog and in emails. I read all of them and they inspire me to keep going. I received my blood work back. Nothing major found, low iron, low hemoglobin, low hematocrit, low MCH, and MCHC and high RDW and MPV levels. Also, high D-Dimer level a coagulation blood marker. My sed rate too was high. This information was for my nurse readers! May sound like a lot…but all should be fixable with supplements for the most part. The question remains…why? Why are these markers out of range? Is it a leaky gut or an absorption issue? Other? Interesting questions to ponder and more testing needs to be done. I would explain each term but don't want to bore the rest of you! Check out terms online for more details if interested. All this testing and poking, prodding and sample collection Ugh! This reminds me with each test, I am an instrument of God's peace. I will do whatever I can to help those that come after me with this disease. I will do whatever it takes to assist in finding contributing factors and solutions for those with ALS.

Thank goodness my cavitation surgery is over! I had cavitation surgery on my lower left jaw, cleaned and scraped the area where my wisdom teeth once were. My left ear and speech changes were my first noticeable symptoms something was going on. I must say I felt instant relief of pressure and didn't have the need to clench my teeth after the surgery. Prior to the surgery I had ozone shots and an ozone wash where the surgical area was. In addition, I also had ozone shots externally along my neck for lymph node drainage and shots along my scapular area which has really atrophied. Post-surgery for 4 weeks I will continue the ozone shots, continue detoxification homeopathies, take garlic tabs and now an iron supplement and folate due to my blood results. In addition, I have an oral rise containing: calendula and arnica and plantago. In the meantime, I had a follow up visit with Dr. Neuenschwander. He is part of the bioenergy center in Ann Arbor. He utilizes alternative treatments where applicable. He has homeopathic medicine specialists, energy medicine, acupuncture, IV and ozone therapies, etc. He's also started treating viruses with UVLrx ultraviolet light intravenous therapy...I may be up for this next. You can check it out online. It's presently under first step approval from our FDA. Then STEM cell adventures to follow. Now that we have taken care of gut health (ketogenic diet, probiotics and supplements), oral health (amalgam filling removal, cavitation surgery) and metal toxicity... onto other stuff to investigate...possibly a "stealth" pathogen, as derived from some of my blood work. We may entertain the UVLrx therapy for this along with continued hyperbaric oxygen therapy. (I love hyperbaric treatments. This infusion of oxygen in every cell of mine makes me feel in a good way that I ran a marathon but didn't have to sweat! Although exhausting Hyperbaric treatments also make my skin look amazing! No wrinkles...

I have friends contemplating Hyperbaric treatments for anti-aging purposes!) Lol. I'm still walking but getting much more help with showers, dressing, food prep…due to the atrophy in my neck and scapular area both arms are weak and affected. I continue to be surrounded by help and blessed with support. Well thanks for listening and praying. I'll keep you posted. Here's to hoping for a snow day for the kids of Petoskey tomorrow!

Funny stuff to share and a twist of reality.

Journal entry by MaryFran Kolp — 2/6/2016

I often tell my girlfriends…seriously…If I look like I have bed head, or something in my teeth or spots on my shirt please fix it!!! My upper body is now so weak help is not only appreciated but necessary! As many of you can imagine, it's been difficult accepting help. Andy and my Frantabulous Friends are all angels. I am so grateful. Words are simply not enough. I now have Andy bath me, my Frantabulous Friends dress and pull up my drawers also a special thanks to Chanin Spadafore and her staff at La Dolce Vita Salon in Petoskey. They donate their time and service to me weekly and my family. Please consider them in Petoskey for your families' hair care and nail and skin care needs. They are very gracious and professional! I again have difficulties with help and service, but I've learned to look at this a special way. Those of you that have followed the "Downtown Abby" series, I've quit the self-pity of needing help and simply pretend I'm like a queen or like "Mary" from the series, waited on, dressed, made meals, driven everywhere… I bet Mary even had Anna pluck the unwanted hairs on her chin! The other day I asked a friend to help me rid the few coarse hairs that show up monthly on me! We laughed she couldn't see them! Ha-ha! All my friends are at the beginning of bifocal stage or in the middle of it and they can't see them either! Ha-ha! As for health updates, I actually look good…with my slim frame I either look like Twiggy (a model from the 60's) or an Ethiopian! Nevertheless, I don't need to drop weight for spring break this year! Also, I'm continuing ozone treatments, hyperbaric and acupuncture! I still do some physical therapy and walk daily. I'm undergoing more testing…blood work and other excreted body waste. Next steps include possible Ultraviolet light therapy and then more testing and revisiting STEM cell stuff. Day by day is how we're doing it!

Danny and Megan are doing great in school and athletics! Meg's basketball season is done. The girls did well 11-9, not bad for a rebuilding year. Meg is now fully engrossed with travel AAU volleyball out of Midland! They are climbing up and ranked 12th out of 50 in their division! We travel every other weekend for tournaments until mid-June! The Petoskey Northman Varsity went undefeated in their BNC conference this year. Districts start in a week! Good luck Northmen! Danny had a great season with this special group of 11 seniors! As for Andy he's cutting back on work to help more at home. All is good! Keep the prayers coming! Hugs and blessings to all of you!

Petoskey Northmen had a great season !
Journal entry by MaryFran Kolp — 3/11/2016

A 20-2 season and a conference championship are nothing to be bummed about! Unfortunately, the streak came to an end at Traverse City West High school against TC West. We lost 68-60. We were down by 15 at halftime, honestly TC West played real well. We came within 4 but didn't break away. The 11 seniors were amazing and great leaders. Danny learned a lot. Danny played well and a lot tonight. He had a great learning season. Now we're off to Waterford, MI for Megan's travel volleyball with the Midland team this weekend. Then Danny starts travel AAU basketball. Keep moving forward, learn from life lessons and always be grateful. Have a great weekend! Remember God's always got your back!

Megan's 16U Midland AAU team Champions!
Journal entry by MaryFran Kolp — 3/13/2016

Success this weekend! The 16U Midland team, of which Meg is a part, won in the 18U open Gold bracket! We are so proud of the girls they played way over-the-top!!! Thank you, Mike & Shelly Davis, Carl & Carol Kolp, Doug, Tracy, Nathan, Madeline and Nora Skene, Uncle Bob Gurzick and Josh & Natalie, Sydney and Ethan Reed!!! I'm sure our cheering session helped with win!

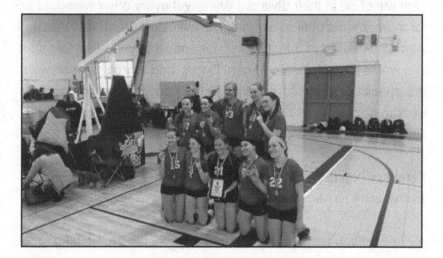

Happy Easter to all!!!
Journal entry by MaryFran Kolp — 3/23/2016

Warning this is the longest entry yet! Forgive me but lots to share! This Lenten and Easter season has been most interesting for me this year. This season has been about sacrifice, offering, service, hope and renewal. Previous years I have offered help, service and encouraged and practiced sacrifice. It's been almost 2 years since my diagnosis, since then I've grown in my Faith and I've been the recipient of divine interventions. It's an odd feeling being the one in need of help. Family, friends, church members, community members and strangers have all stepped up to help my family and me. Friends and family have driven our kids to their AAU basketball and volleyball events. I've tried to express my heartfelt gratitude and appreciation, but my word choices don't do justice to my true feelings. This journey has been terrible at moments mostly because of the fear of the unknown. Daily slowly slipping away, my freedoms to drive, self-dress, coming and going as I please and drinking a cappuccino with one hand…all ending. BUT God has surrounded me with warriors! Those that drive me, accompany me, dress me and assist with cappuccino consumption!!! There you have it…like all situations is your cup half full or half empty? God gives us that choice and we get to pick!

We're looking forward to spring break as a family. Heading to San Diego, hanging at the beach with the Collins family very dear friends. I'm looking forward to quality time with Jeff, Mel, and my "other son and daughter" Hunter and Kira! In addition, I'll be having my first consultant with doctors in California regarding STEM cell treatment and what's entailed. Thanks to many of you for the possibility to start this process through gifts and fundraising done so far. As many of you know many treatments, including this experimental procedure, are costly and not covered by insurance. But, crossing off the list, things that are not systematically balanced in me is a process. If we can gain any answers from my case for future recipients of this ALS beast…we should do it!

Recently I had more blood work and other testing done. My blood work indicated I'm hormonally deficient therefore I'm now on natural compounded thyroid, progesterone, testosterone and DHEA supplements. Iron infusion is being investigated too, as these levels are deficient. As for my lung capacity this is surprisingly pretty good and efficient! Often with ALS patients breathing and swallowing become issues. I apparently am not there yet! Another interesting to note, it's been over a month since my amalgam fillings extractions and my urine assessment indicates my metal toxins are down. We're now on to treat something else. I am still continuing hyperbaric oxygen treatments whenever I go downstate for the kids AAU events. My body responds great to this treatment. I love oxygen! In addition, following my last treatment, I will share I also did an "anal ozone" treatment. The patient, me, simply places a small tube with a hole in it in the rectum and ozone is then slowly and a small amount infused. I only mention this because after this treatment I had an immediate positive response. I had no fasciculations and no twitching for about 8 hours after the treatment. It has been a long time since I felt this way. Normal...no twitching. I even was able to drive half way home from downstate after this treatment. Therefore, I felt it was worth noting. Since this response, being the researcher, I am...I did it again and had again a similar response. Now I'm looking to purchase this unit for home use. Small expense for the benefit. There have been suggestions that a virus may contribute to ALS, at least in part. Therefore, I will be starting IVLrx...IV light therapy, there has been some research in other countries utilizing this therapy. Many pathogens and viruses are so difficult to get rid of. The thought is if you don't rid or dismantle the pathogen... What good can STEM cell treatment do if the element still causing the body distress is present? This is why this is such a tricky process. It would be great if it was so easy as taking a pill to fix this, or simply have STEM cells infused in my spine to be fixed. But we all know it's not that simple! Again, there are no guarantees! What do I have to lose?

You see my ALS symptoms may be associated with my gut health. To find out more about how many diseases, especially neurological problems may have a direct correlation with gut health consider a couple of reads. "Brain Maker" by Dr. David Perlmutter, "Medical Medium" by Anthony Williams. Focusing more intensely on gut health is my medical team's plan.

I may have shared more then you ever cared to know but others with ALS have been reading and following this blog. In traditional medicine many with ALS are not given hope. There is still so much to do and explore. One day at a time. Don't leave any stone unturned! Happy Easter! Don't lose the magic of this Holy season! Keep on going! Spring is here! God bless each and every one of you!

ALS friends and those with neurological disorders
Journal entry by MaryFran Kolp — 4/2/2016

I have been asked on numerous occasions after my last two blogs to share what supplements I'm on. I've shared this and deep detail in earlier blogs. Please note you should discuss with your health professional before taking supplements. I have had many tests...Lyme disease, muscle enzyme testing, heavy metal testing, gut health testing, hormones, bacterial, fungus, viruses all investigated. I have had bloodwork, urine and fecal testing and retesting to determine my regimen. But in summary I am newly on progesterone, testosterone, and an estrogen supplement (I am 48 at that age with a lot of changes going on) after my last round of blood work. The following supplements I've been on the following for quite some time: CoQ10, Inosine, neo40, magnesium citrate, magnesium taurate, iron, ferrion, nrf2 activator, DHA, DHEA, garlic, vitamin D drops. Specifically, for gut health, commensil probiotics, Restore and HPL probiotic are taken before meals. Additional support, A-akg powder, L-serine powder, and Trehalose. I also continue to get a B12 shot twice a week and take oral liposomal glutathione. In addition, once a week I get an IV which includes magnesium, vitamin C, vitamin B and some homeopathies. Lastly, I still do hyperbaric treatments when I'm downstate and ozone treatments too. Obviously, some care is rationed due to cost. These above-mentioned treatments and acupuncture are added when possible. In addition, I've been blessed with Orthosport, specifically Shelly Budnick for PT massages and H wave treatments. And, Rae, a dear friend, from Petoskey Hand Therapy for her personal help with stretching and exercises. Never underestimate prayer too! I've received the blessed sacrament Anointing of the Sick. Thank God for my Faith. Also, newly added, I've purchased an ozone machine. This has an immediate impact on me. It really makes me feel calm and relaxed, no muscle twitching! Lastly, consider a Paleo or ketogenic diet. Work with a licensed professional on diet...but thus far I believe diet has had a major impact on my neurological disorder and symptoms. For support start with any of Dr. David Perlmutter's books..."Grain Brain" could be helpful. Sounds like a lot I know, and it is. It's a full-time job! But, if we can get some answers who knows what we'll discover. Hope this helps and answers general questions you may have on why after 2 years... I'm still walking.

Michigan Mustang's 16 AAU Basketball tournament Champions

Journal entry by MaryFran Kolp — 4/4/2016

This past weekend the boys from the Mustangs won their tournament at the Hype center in Dearborn! Great tournament! Nice win! Congratulations to Danny, Tray, Davion, Xavion, Gabe, Goliath, Luke, Tanner, Jacob and Taylor!

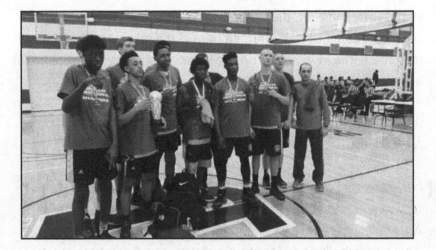

In California at Dr. Steenblock's office
Journal entry by MaryFran Kolp — 4/7/2016

It's hard for me to believe California has drought problems! Our first two days in San Diego it was 60 degrees and rain! Ugh! Well I guess if I'm visiting doctors it's good not to be too warm or sunny out. Just feel bad for the kids! Meg's bummed to be tan less…but it may be a blessing no skin cancer!

My visit with Dr Steenblock was beneficial. I have more testing that needs to be done. More blood, fecal and urine tests but looking first at virus, bacterial and fungal components. First, he feels I have gut issues associated with my ALS. So, we'll get a further assessment on what's going on there. Then entertain STEM cell interventions.

Our spring break ended up being a great visit! We were able to spend quality time with the Collins family! Surfing, eating, drinking and college touring! We too were blessed to see the Hogen family, the Murphy family, the Danly family and some summer Lake Charlevoix friends! What a treat! Everyone is doing well, and the kids are all growing up! Also, we had a great visit with Sarah and Ken, dear friends that did a little shopping with our kids! Meg and Dan were so happy! It was so nice to catch up and see some loved ones on the west coast! It was a great trip in all. We even had sunshine the last few days!

A great Mother's Day wish to all!
Journal entry by MaryFran Kolp — 5/8/2016

I do hope the snow is behind us for a while! Happiest of Mother's Day to you and your Moms! Our kids are well! Meg busy with AAU volleyball every weekend until early June, Danny busy with AAU basketball. Andy leaves his group, so he can help me more June 15th. He will then become an independent consultant and work as it works out for our family. He isn't retiring, just getting a little more flexibility with his schedule. Andy's partners and their families have been so supportive and gracious, we can't thank them enough. A special thank you to all my caregivers. The needs for help are increasing and at every turn you are there with love, humor, respect and genuine care. Divine interventions keep me going.

This past month a bitter sweet happening… I'm no longer driving, and we traded my Traverse for a Ford Flex…I call the Gangster car. Although not the most attractive in my opinion, it is very comfortable and spacious for travel, especially for tall families. Nevertheless, bittersweet… I'm now officially chauffeured… Kind of like the movie "Driving Miss Daisy". Mom's and Dad's treasure carpooling and carting kids around, no matter how hectic, you never know when you may not have this gift any longer!

Next steps for my treatment include more testing… I consider my body a test tube, (hopefully we can get more information to defeat this disease with my soul intact of course! A twist of Ultraviolet light therapy, Colposcopy upcoming… Then STEM cell prep (not embryonic)! I'll keep you posted! Hugs to you and your families! I'm so blessed for your help, prayers and positivity! Blessings sent to all of you!

Silver bracket champions in the premium division

Journal entry by MaryFran Kolp — 5/9/2016

Congratulations Michigan Elite Diamond 16u team! Champions again!

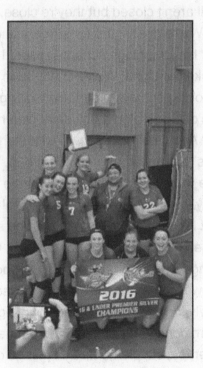

Update from the Kolp family

Journal entry by MaryFran Kolp — 5/21/2016

I pray this greets all of you doing well this beautiful spring! The Kolps are hanging in there! We have had some great moments and we have had some challenging ones. Megan's volleyball team continues to improve and do excellent in their tournament play winning a lot! We're so proud of Megan's team and Megan she has just excelled and grown so much as a young lady and in the sport! One week until the state competition in Grand Rapids! Wish us luck! As for Danny, we have had an unfortunate setback, Danny has torn his tendon affiliated with his knee cap again. He was scrimmaging when it happened. He was 6'4 at his last knee surgery he's now 6'8 two years later, this may be part of it. His growth plates still aren't closed but they're close. So, his summer season is done. We're gearing up for surgery and with a little luck he'll be ready for his junior high school season! I have to believe God has our backs but Ugh!!! We've cried, been sad, even angry but now we're moving on day by day. Reminding ourselves daily it's a small piece of God's plan a universal plan not just about the Kolps! As for Andy, he's gearing up with starting his own business as he is leaving his existing ER group. He will begin locums mid-June while taking a big chunk of the summer off to be with our family. He's fishing again and biking! I miss doing this with him, but I'm so glad he's back to doing some things for him! As for me I need more help these days. God's easing me into this change with friends and family support. Often both arms don't work well, often friends and family assist me in eating these days. Slowly losing freedoms and counting my blessings along the way. I'm continuing with ozone treatment, acupuncture, physical therapy, supplements and just go day by day. I'm not going to die anytime soon, so don't be alarmed. But, if I pass from ALS please don't put in print anywhere I lost my battle with this disease. I hate how they do that with those that had cancer and die! This disease has shown me many fruits of my volunteering and interactions with people! I've even grown closer to my Frantabulous Friends having discussions I never would have had if I wasn't sick! So, however gruesome this gets, as I'm sure it may. I have some great experiences and I've gotten to know many of my acquaintances as good friends. We spend quality time together often. The kind of friends that feed ya, bath you and laugh and cry with you …without judging me. I never would have been blessed with these gifts! Also, crying I now view as cleansing the soul! After a good cry I feel better and lighter! Don't you? How has crying been viewed as a weakness when it's so powerful! Switching gears…

Many of you know last evening was the 25th Anniversary of the St. Francis Gala Auction. Katie and Amy did a great job as chairpersons this year for this event. Last evening, as I sat at a table filled with friends and surrounding our table were more friends! One of my, thought to be, worse nightmares came true, I was fed my dinner at a formal event! I had Andy on one side and my friend Vanessa on the other, not missing a beat and scooping in bite after bite. But, I survived as did they. Clean plate and no food on my dress!!! As I looked around this table I was awestruck by the friendships that shared this table and those nearby. As the Lord knows we all have issues, I witnessed laughter, tears, concern and elated spirits as we had the $20,000 raffle ticket winner at our table! Congratulations Mike and Lanette Hoffman! What an evening with special men and women surrounding us! Our angels on earth! Enjoy this beautiful Michigan spring! I am!

Summer vacation is here! What a crazy start!
Journal entry by MaryFran Kolp — 6/17/2016

Truth is Stranger Than Fiction! The Kolp family summer vacation is off with a Great bang, exams are done, snow is gone, summer activities have begun! The Kolp kids are rocking! Megan had a spectacular travel AAU volleyball season! Collegiate basketball recruiting has begun for Danny! This blog I'll update you on the kids. Then next entry immediately following I'll update you on my health stuff and treatment.

This past June 15th the NCAA guidelines permit college coaches to contact perspective college basketball athletes from the class of 2018. All of which Danny is part of this class and is ranked in the top 100 for the class of 2018 for basketball recruits. Although we must be honest, since the knee cap ligament injury we weren't sure with missing the summer AAU basketball season who or if anyone would call Danny as a prospective recruit. We were pleasantly surprised and so happy for Danny. On the 15th at midnight he received a tweet from coach Smith from Central Michigan University confirming their offer for a basketball scholarship. In addition, he received another offer from the University of Toledo. This was followed by numerous phone calls of interest from Iowa, Duquesne, University of Milwaukee, Oakland University, Air force, and DePaul! Calls are still coming in forgive me if I missed a few. Danny's phone is "blowing up"! And, despite Danny's injury, Coach Beilein from the University of Michigan called, and Coach Dan Fife from Michigan State came to visit Danny at MSU Team camp yesterday. We were so happy for Danny, as he was very concerned that he wouldn't get any calls due to his injury and missing most of the summer basketball season. Please pray for him! Especially this Monday that God has his hand in Danny's surgery scheduled at Beaumont Royal Oak, with Danny, his physician and nurses and techs. Andy and I could use a few too!

Megan's AAU volleyball season was a great success! Her coach is in the process of creating a recruiting video for her. It's hard to believe but Megan may actually know where she's going to college before Danny! Volleyball recruiting works this way, early verbal commitments are common. Although she's only 14, she's already being looked at 3.9 GPA, smart and 6'2 working on her vertical jump and foot speed she's something to reckon with and willing to work very hard to maximize her potential. It's not easy finding a 6'2 coordinated young lady and she's all that!

Our kids, as all of you know have had a few rough years with my health issues. Andy and I are so proud of them and thank all of you for nurturing their God given gifts. We tell the kids often to those that are given much will be asked for in return. They have been blessed by YOU and me! They're fighters and despite obstacles they're doing their thing, and well day by day!

Happy 50th Anniversary Dan & Carole Peterlin
Journal entry by MaryFran Kolp — 6/22/2016

It's hard to believe 50 years!!! Congratulations Mom and Dad! I pray you have many more fruitful years ahead of you! If all of you reading this could offer my folks a prayer and good wishes on their special day that would be great! Thursday, June 23rd! It seems like yesterday we had a 25th Anniversary party, and I thought that was a long time! Now Andy and I have been married 20 years and have two teenagers! Crazy how time flies! No party this time but we'll do a small dinner at my sister Natalie's cottage over the fourth! They are wonderful parents! Natalie and I have learned a lot from their love and example! Great human beings, parents and friends. We love you both so much! A priest once told my folks…a good marriage is not the wedding day but 50 years from that day and witnessing all your loved ones and blessings you've accrued over the years!!! You have a lot of blessings! God gave me the two of you! We are so grateful and blessed!!!

Moving forward…one doctor at a time!
Journal entry by MaryFran Kolp — 7/16/2016

The past few weeks have been nonstop for the Kolps! My birthday was very special this year, we celebrated as a family my parent's 50th anniversary, my birthday and that I'm still walking after being diagnosed with ALS 2 years ago. Danny's still on the mend, a real trooper he hates not being active during this healing process. He has 2 more weeks in his brace but has been doing some upper body weights. Megan attended a team camp at Grand Valley State University for volleyball! They did well, 3rd overall! She then immediately went to elite volleyball camp at the University of Michigan. She loved camp and enjoyed her cousin Sydney as her roommate! Andy is on sabbatical while we figure out our family plan. However, it hasn't been all rest, caring for Danny and me. In addition, Andy started his business during this time. He's an independent contractor now and many calls are coming in for work. He'll be back in ER's in August while accommodating our family needs too. He has been amazing caring for us, never complaining with our requests. As for my health it's getting more challenging, but God always puts an angel in my presence to get me through. Whether I receive a card a call or a friendly hug or prayers! While downstate I met with an eye doctor, Dr. Debby Feinberg that placed prisms in my eyeglass prescription, it appears I may have had an injury to my head or neck, or trauma sometime in my life probably through athletics. I can't believe the clarity and steadiness a pair of glasses can give me. Through this appointment Dr. Debby recommended I consult with another neurologist that "thinks outside the box" I was impressed with Integrated Neurologist Dr. Giressh Velugubonti's assessment process, evaluation and then his treatment which concluded I needed to be on some antiviral meds, antibiotics and detox following extensive bloodwork too. And pursuing stem cells were all once again put in play. It appears I will be getting Stem cell treatment Mid-August. We're working through details. Lastly, I met with an integrative nutritionist while downstate. Aarti Batavia, her training was done with Dr. Perlmutter and his nutrition professionals. Healing with food can't hurt in my desire to be more well! When given the cards I've been dealt, you choose sole "evidence based traditional medicine" and while "no cause and no cure for ALS" you simply report every 6 months as you progress or become part of a study where I would be taken off supplements and put on a placebo or drug...or you look at alternatives. Pulling from all areas of science to Methodically create a new path? I like Physicians that think "outside the box" and pray others with ALS seek other treatments. If it doesn't cure them it can make one feel better! God willing if I get well or stable I'll be pushing for research and treatment coverage of alternative means for people with ALS.

July 19, 2016

MaryFran had a Mediator Release Test. It basically showed which foods and additives she had reactions to and should probably avoid. She strongly reacted to green peppers, mint, kaput, pistachio, mango, and soybean. She moderately reacted to almond, American cheese, apple, baker's yeast, broccoli, celery, cheddar, yellow 5, grape, honeydew, lettuce, mushroom, mustard, orange, oregano, papaya, quinoa, sole, string bean, and yellow squash. In the summary, it says that if you have previously regularly consumed before testing and not had any allergic, autoimmune, or other inflammation-provoking or symptom-provoking reaction, they are probably okay to ingest.

Stem cell treatment scheduled
Journal entry by MaryFran Kolp — 8/6/2016

As this spectacular summer comes to an end, fall sports begin and cutting-edge medical procedures attempted... Andy and I will be heading to California to begin a 2-week stem cell treatment for me. If you're interested in learning more about stem cells check out http://dld-conference.com/events/stem cells -the- future

-of-Medicine. It's a 20-minute video that explains what stem cells are, how they may be key to the future of medicine and there's an example of an ALS case showing improvement. This process slightly modified, as my stem cells will be extracted from my hip bones, as I do not have much body fat. I will begin at noon on August 22nd in San Clemente, CA luckily not too far from friends in Laguna Hills, where we will be staying. Another divine intervention, the Hogan and Danley families helping us when we're out there. In this stretch before stem cells, I had some more blood work done. Another Lyme's Western blot test that came back with a few positive bands but nothing conclusive to standards. In addition, I tested positive for relapsing fever, a spirochete-bacteria, a cousin to Lyme. Therefore, my supplement and prescription has changed in this stretch before stem cells. I am now on heavy antibiotics, antiviral medication and 2 antifungals. Reason for the antifungal's research shows in autopsies 100% of ALS patients have Candida overgrowth in the brain. So, we'll have done a lot of the ground work prior to stem cells based on the limited research available regarding this disease. This includes: dietary restrictions, supplements and prescriptions, detoxification for metals, amalgam filling removal, hyperbaric treatments, ozone treatments, acupuncture, cranial sacral therapy, multiple doctors' visits and numerous prayers! Much not covered by insurance. All this in hopes STEM cell treatment may halt my disease or help and improve my symptoms. No guarantees. Lastly, I can't thank enough Robin and Barry Bennett, the steel drum band and all of our friends making this ALS fundraiser for us on Tuesday, at the Rose Garden, at the Perry Hotel possible. I don't even know who to thank there are so many of you Angels! We are humbled and grateful.

A Glimpse of Heaven in Northern Michigan!
Journal entry by MaryFran Kolp — 8/11/2016

I was humbled and very grateful for all the teenagers of the Petoskey Steel Drum Band, the instructors Mr. Bennett and Mr. Ryan and a special thanks to Mr. Harvey for MC'ing this event. You all haven't only built a spectacular band program but have been instrumental in the development of numerous young teens into leaders and strong contributors to society! Amazing program! Thanks to all of the donors, the Angels that helped with the event, especially Deanna Beaudoin who stepped up to be in charge in the last hours, and Robin Bennett who from a conversation in La Dolce Vita, our local amazing salon...she said she's doing a fund-raiser for our cause...and made it happen. It was a very successful event both spirituality and financially. Even our kids had friends present. Megan's teammates from travel volleyball in Midland came to the event to surprise and support her! Financially close to $35,000 was raised and McLaren Northern Michigan Foundation picked up our flights! That's crazy money and support. Awesome community! Seriously no words to summarize the feelings or gratitude. While many of you know my supplements, alternative treatments aren't covered by insurance. This stem cell treatment truly would have financially put Andy over the edge! But God provides and many of you were his angels doing his work for me, and hopefully many others to come. I pray this stem cell treatment has a positive effect! My intention is to write a book entitled "Divine Interventions" or "Restarting your Nervous System." Time will tell! We will see. Andy and I are departing in an hour. I report at noon at the clinic tomorrow! I will keep you posted through this blog. Extra prayers welcome! Thank you everyone for everything! Make it a great day!!!

Stem cells extracted and starting to process
Journal entry by MaryFran Kolp — 8/23/2016

A special thank you to our friends and hosts, Bob and Trudy Hogan! They have a beautiful over the top home and are allowing us to stay during this process. We are so blessed, they live 20 minutes from the clinic! After a physical day one and some supportive IV's, day 2 brought a bone marrow extraction from my hip. Extracting 7 "turkey baster full" (60ml), 300ml of bone marrow, containing stem cells. 4 immediately infused in me via IV. 2 are being treated with umbilical cord blood (not embryonic) containing growth factors and stem cells that will be nurtured and injected into specific areas in my spine over the week, predominantly the neck area. I also will continue Infrared treatments, hypoxia therapy, shots and hyperbaric to increase stem cell proliferation. Everyone is very kind! Wanted to give an update! I feel your prayers! Sorry this is short but I'm exhausted! Love you all!

Beginning of week 2
Journal entry by MaryFran Kolp — 8/29/2016

If anyone gets a chance, please wish Megan a happy 15th birthday today! Well, we've begun week 2 of our stem cell treatments! I had another 300 mL of stem cells and bone marrow extracted this time from my right hip. I am exhausted but feel as if progress is being made so I will continue on the journey. I have more infrared light treatments, hyperbaric treatments, shots, and pokes and resubmission of stem cells to look forward to in this upcoming week. I am starting to look forward to coming home as I really miss my kids. Just thinking about them gets me through! Andy has been amazing and a real trooper as I have not been the best of patients! In between all of the pokes and prods we have had some quick little exploration trips investigating Dana Point,

Laguna Hills, and Newport Beach. This is a very beautiful area and we are blessed to be here. I thank you for your continued prayers! They are heartfelt and carrying me through this process. In turn, I have had a lot of downtime and have spent a lot of time praying for each of you; especially those that have commented via text, email or on this Caring Bridge blog!

Home and healing!
Journal entry by MaryFran Kolp — 9/7/2016

As many of you can imagine life has been a whirlwind these past two weeks! It's good to be home, see the kids and get them prepared for another school year. We are so grateful for all of the help and assistance while we were away thank-you to our parents and to Sarah for staying with the kids! Friends, thanks for the food and Gina the blueberry bunt cake! Our experience at Dr. Steenblock's Clinic was very interesting! He has an excellent staff! Hopefully within 3 to 5 weeks we will start seeing some changes from the stem cells that have been cared for and put back into my system. So sorry for the delay in updating this blog, however after my spinal tap I once again had a headache and have been recuperating from that. I'll let you know when I'm ready to have guests! I look forward to filling all of you in on the details of my experience once I'm feeling a little better. Keep the prayers coming! I hope all is well with you and your family! Will look forward to talking soon!

I'm almost back on the grid!
Journal entry by MaryFran Kolp — 9/12/2016

This journey of getting stem cells has been quite an adventure to say the least. I'm back on the grid! If you, and your household, are healthy come on over! I need to try to remain healthy to allow my stem cells to grow most effectively and efficiently! I've missed all of you, but really needed the rest and alone time. Marie kindly created great signs for outside our front door and the garage so if dropping by you'll know if we're up for guests. Thanks Marie! I'm working on sharing some pictures of my experience in California, but my fingers have slowed so I don't text as fast! I wanted to wish my Dad, Dan Peterlin a happy birthday!!! He is the best Dad ever! He was so into us kids, we're so blessed! He would even come watch our games and then have to go back to work after! What Dad does that? We love you Dad!

Infrared therapy
Journal entry by MaryFran Kolp — 9/29/2016

Infrared light therapy stimulates stem cells. The socks on my feet also offered gentle pulses that also may stimulate stem cell growth. I also had an oxygen mask on to control my saturation levels to stimulate again stem cells. I would lay there daily for an hour during my two weeks in California at the clinic.

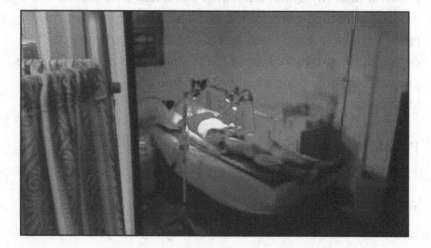

October update

Journal entry by MaryFran Kolp — 10/10/2016

The Kolp kids are doing great! Danny's physical therapy for his knee is progressing nicely as expected and we hope to have him back at basketball by Christmas break. He just finished an official visit to Central Michigan University watching the basketball team practice and the football game and a volleyball match! Great experience! Looking to visit the University of Toledo and Loyola and DePaul Universities soon. Megan has been doing a phenomenal job in volleyball. She is in the local newspaper weekly. It's exciting to see her coming into her own. Unfortunately, in gym class she sprained her foot and was out of commission for a couple of weeks. She will be back for districts this weekend. Andy is doing well he's actually back to work now working about 5 shifts a month at McLaren at this point. Andy went bowhunting for a couple of days downstate with his buddy Randy. A well-deserved break! As for me I feel a little more rested since treatments in California but not much. The progression of muscle weakness has persisted. My arms don't work really well nor do my hands, but I still remain positive and grateful. Daily I'm reminded of the prayers and support we have. Seriously, I have so many great friends surrounding me in my home and at games! I envision this being like a glimpse of Heaven. Julie, Kim, Lynn, Maggie, Pam, Pat, Lanette and Gina all around me while watching my baby girl play volleyball! Total Heaven here on earth for me! Remember to celebrate every day! It's becoming harder and harder to type but I will do this blog as long as I can. It just may take me a little longer than previously. Because I don't write anymore those of you suffering I would have sent cards but since I am unable to do so just know that you are in our thoughts and prayers. I know many of you reading this have struggles of your own. My card to you is please look up on YouTube the song by Casting Crowns "Just be held". I think of you Rose Heiler, Gail Meloche, Brenda Meloche, Jerry Weurding, Bob and Doris Baker, Paula Chilcote, Jeff Cech, Elliot, Klimas, and Lukas families!! Those of us suffering I asked but you offered up your discomfort to some of my fellow ALS friends: Ken Miller who is presently receiving a similar treatment that I did at the same location in California. Also, if you can pray for Tammy Pawlowski and Amy Janisse! I love you all!

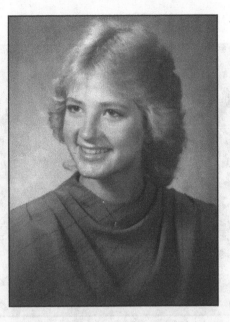

Senior class photo, class of 1985

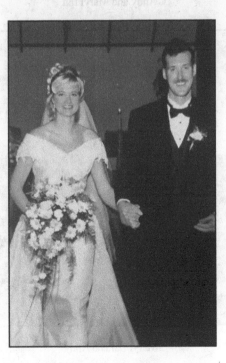

Their wedding day

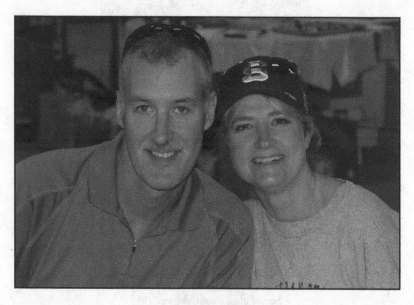

Andy and MaryFran

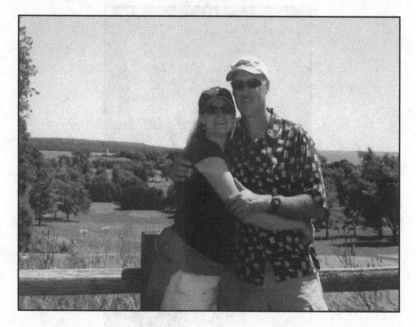

MaryFran and Andy

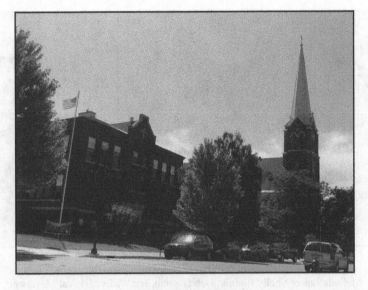

St. Francis Xavier School

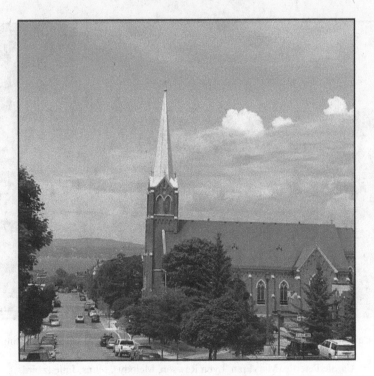

St. Francis Xavier Church

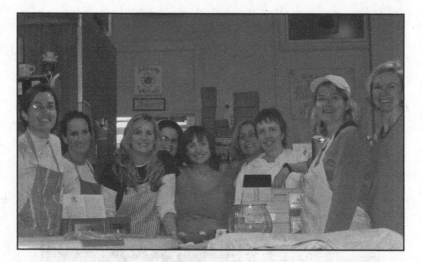

Some early members of the Organic Cooking Club—Maggie Kromm, Melinda Eaton, Shelly Budnik, Deb Gagnon, Jen Waldvogel, Val Meyerson, Julie Adams, MaryFran Kolp, and Marie Law

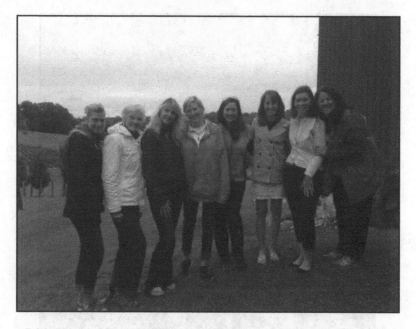

Celebrating MaryFran's birthday a day early—and a day before her devastating diagnosis; in the picture are MaryFran's sister Natalie Reed, her mother Carole Peterlin, MaryFran, Lynn Rawson, Melody Collins, Julie Izzard, Kathy Coveyou, and Lanette Hoffman.

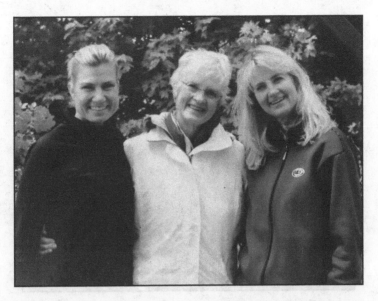

Natalie Peterlin Reed, Carole Peterlin, and MaryFran Peterlin Kolp

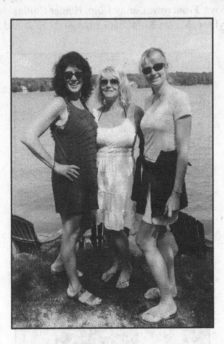

Kim Wroblewski, Deanna Beaudoin, and MaryFran at Deanna's home.
It was about a month after her diagnosis. We met for lunch and Deanna wanted
to tell Fran about a book she found about care groups. Little did we know
how this meeting would change our lives forever.

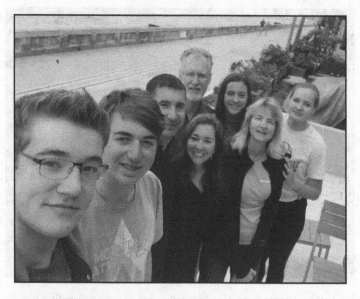

The Collins and Kolp families have been close friends since they met in Lamaze class pregnant with the boys. Front row: Danny Kolp, Hunter Collins, Jeff Collins, Melody Collins, MaryFran, Megan Kolp. Back row: Andy Kolp and Kira Collins.

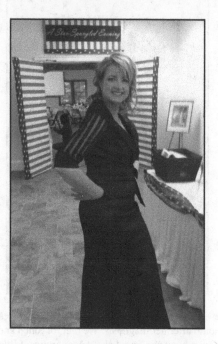

MaryFran chairing the school auction.

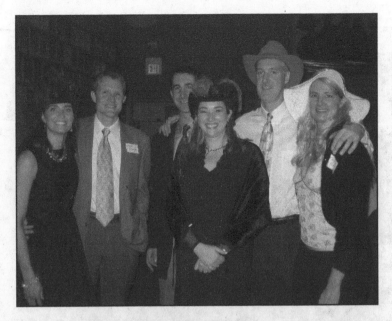

St. Francis Gala Auction fun! Some years we had themes. Above, the theme was
Kentucky Derby. Left to right are Maggie and Jason Kromm, Jeff and
Melody Collins, and Andy and MaryFran Kolp.

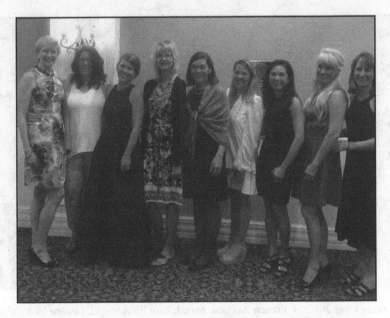

Left to right: Marie Law, Lanette Hoffman, Kim Scholl, MaryFran,
Kathy Coveyou, Jennifer Buck, Vanessa Ceniza, Beth Burke, and Julie Izzard

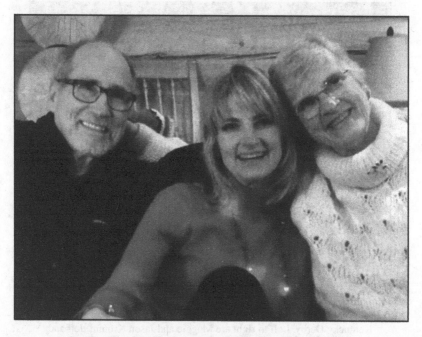

Dan Peterlin, MaryFran, and Carole Peterlin, Christmas 2014

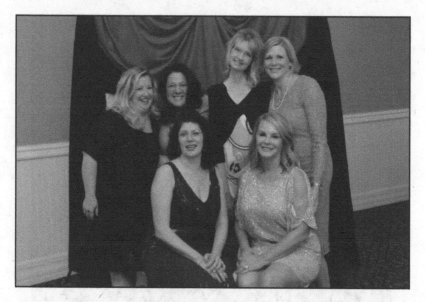

Spring Fling 2017, St. Francis Auction; seated: Kim Wroblewski, Deanna Beaudoin;
back row: Lisa Pulaski, Lanette Hoffman, MaryFran Kolp, and Lynn Rawson

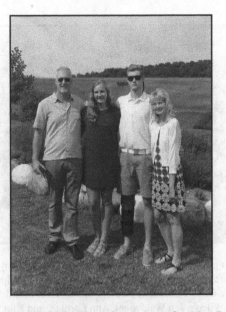

Andy, Megan, Danny, and MaryFran about a year after MaryFran's diagnosis

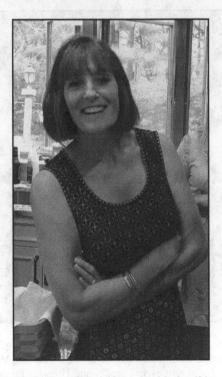

Terri Kolp Reynolds, the best sister-in-law/friend!

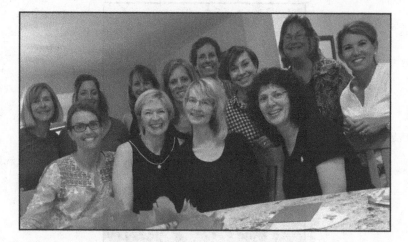

We were celebrating Marie, MaryFran, and Kim's fiftieth birthdays. Pictured on first row, left to right, are Maggie Kromm, Marie Law, MaryFran Kolp, Kim Wroblewski; back row are Cheryl Eberhart, Terri Reynolds, Julie Izzard, Tina Wilder, Joelle Wilcox, Jen Waldvogel, Ann Carolan, and Kim Scholl.

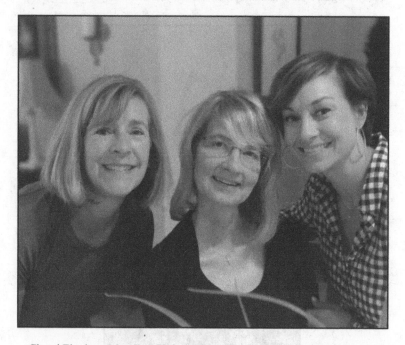

Cheryl Eberhart, MaryFran Kolp, and Jen Waldvogel; Cheryl and Jen were indispensable, along with Terri Reynolds, for bathing MaryFran. They came almost every Tuesday and Thursday for months.

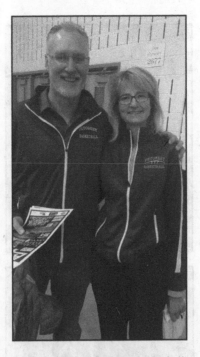

Andy and MaryFran attending a basketball game.

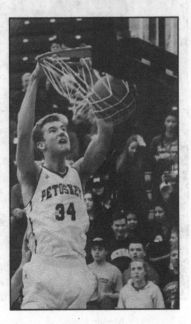

Danny Kolp

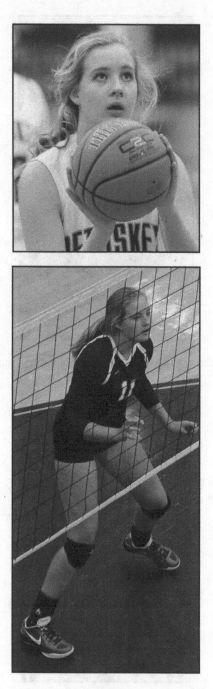

Megan Kolp

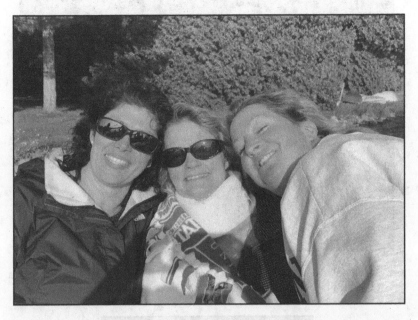

Kim Wroblewski, MaryFran and Lisa Pulaski on our last pontoon boat trip

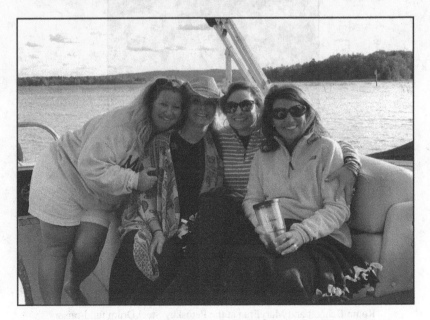

Lisa Pulaski, Deanna Beaudoin, Jennifer Waldvogel and Kim Scholl

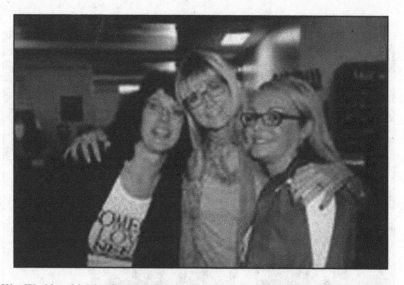

Kim Wroblewski, MaryFran and Deanna Beaudoin at the Strike-Out ALS fund-raiser.
It was the first event of several to help raise money to offset treatment costs.

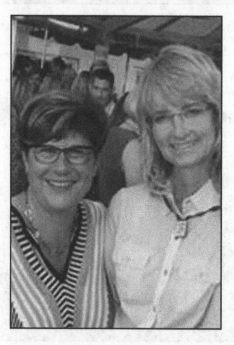

Robin Bennett and MaryFran at the Petoskey Steel Drum fund-raiser.
Robin is married to one of the band directors and a friend of MaryFran.
She was the driving force behind this event.

PART 3

This was the last journal entry that MaryFran was able to do herself. Her voice was getting very weak, so it was difficult for her to voice-text, and she had lost the use of her arms and fingers. I did not know we were going to write this book and regret not starting a journal earlier. The next entries were from her mother's notes interspersed with my own journal entries, which I started in January 2018 every time I visited.

August 14, 2017

MaryFran was prescribed baclofen 10 mg tab, half tab p.o. TID 30 days.

August 26, 2017

MaryFran is consulting with Dr. Velugubanti of Integrative Neurology, PLLC. He has prescribed for her olive leaf extract 1,000 mg for chronic infections. Activated charcoal 560 mg 3× daily 2 hours away from meals, supplements, probiotics, antibiotics, NA-C antivirals. Activated charcoal is for 14 days. Biocidin 5 drops 3× daily for 8 weeks. Interphase plus once daily for 2 months. Then stop supplementation of what is listed above olive leaf and Biocidin and redraw labs five days thereafter, then once labs are obtained then restart supplementation. 5-HTP 100 mg 3× daily.

It was around this time when she finally agreed to a wheelchair. She was still able to walk with someone holding her from behind. The problem was her head and neck muscles were now so weak that she could barely hold her head up. She still remained positive and attended Mass. She always thought that if she could walk, there was still hope.

November 27, 2017

Dr. Velugubanti prescribed Feosol 325 mg 1 tablet BID, Biocidin 5 drops p.o. TID 1 oz/30 ml, Turmeric with black pepper 1 capsule p.o. BID, and olive leaf extract p.o. TID.

November 28, 2017

Carole sent an email to Aarti to let her know that MaryFran has claimed that some of the supplements are making her nauseous. This is causing her to have a loss of appetite and less consumption of food and liquid. They began experimenting with reducing or eliminating each supplement that was determined to cause nausea. Her appetite increased significantly, as also liquid consumption. Testing with a pendulum was used to determine the following.

Supplements testing as needed but causing nausea:
Brain cell support
Acetyl L Carnitine
CoQ10 reduced to one 1× a day
Magnesium reduced to one 1× a day
Ascorbic acid reduced to half scoop 1× a day
NAC

Previously reduced evening primrose ½ tsp 3× a day
Phospotidal choline ½ tsp 3× a day

Supplements testing as not needed and cause nausea:
Berberine plus
NADH

Supplements testing as not needed (but do not cause nausea):
5HTP

Interphase Plus

Saccharomyces boulardii

All other supplements have tested as needed and as not causing nausea.

We will share details and specifics at the Skype conference on Thursday.

Were you forwarded the results of her follow-up blood work on October 13? We will also share information from yesterday's follow-up meeting with Dr. V's staff physician, Srilatha Thadur, M.D. the photos of the prescriptions are attached.

Thanks ahead of time for all that you do.

Carole

December 1, 2017

MaryFran was taking the following vitamins and supplements:

Arabinogalactan Powder ½ tsp. 2× a day

Tru Bifido 1 capsule

B complex 1 capsule 2× a day

Vitamin D 1 capsule

Magnesium 2 capsules 2× a day

Acetyl L Carnitine 1 capsule

Arthdygestzyme 2 capsule 3× a day

Butyrate 2 capsules a day

Brain cell support 1 capsule 2× a day

Ultra-Pure McTail

Barbering Plus 1 capsule 2× a day

Enada NADH-5 1 capsule 2× a day

Vitamin C powder 1 scoop 2× a day

Lipothiamine 1 capsule 2× a day

CoQ10 1 capsule 2× a day

Lipoid Acid 1 capsule 2× a day

LDA Trace Mineral Complex 1 capsule

Glycine Sticks 1 a day

Evening Primrose 1 tsp 3× a day (for menopause)

Phospatidyl Choline 1 tsp 3× a day

Lithium Orotate 1 capsule 1× a day first week, then 1 capsule 2× a day 5 weeks

Neurological Mag 2 capsules 2× a day

Rhodiola Rosea 1 capsule 2× a day

Mitochondrial NRG 2 capsules 2× a day

LVGB Complex with high fat meals

She also gets a B12 injection, melatonin at night.

January of 2018

Her mom found a neurotherapy center. She started having biofeedback sessions with Dr. Spinazola every weekend. This was thought to help decrease anxiety and irritability. Arrangements were made with friends to help get her downstate to Ann Arbor for the treatments. She would stay with her parents and they would also take her to craniosacral massage appointments.

January 10, 2018

Dr. Linkner felt that MaryFran would benefit from drinking Nourish or the trademark name Liquid Hope. Her mom was able to get it covered through the insurance as she was to the point of having difficulty eating solid foods now. This is an organic, functional formularies meal replacement. You need a physician prescription in order to use it. It basically contains vitamins with garbanzo beans, peas, carrots, brown rice, flax oil, sprouted quinoa, sweet potato, broccoli, almond butter, kale, and some spices. One pouch has 450 calories and 23 grams of protein. She keeps losing weight, which is not a good indicator for patients with ALS.

Side note:

Her weight has been steadily decreasing and while for most of us that is usually a good thing, for ALS patients that is bad indicator. From August of 2016 she weighed 122 lbs., and by November of 2017 she was down to 107 lbs.

January 31, 2018

Today was a difficult day. Terri weighed MaryFran and she weighed 98 lbs. She is also very stressed about finances. Having ALS is not cheap. Insurance hardly covers anything. When I came at noon to help, she had been crying quite a bit this morning and was finishing her lunch. She loves to have the massager on her limbs, so I did that. I helped Terri with dishes, laundry, and the mail. I worked on putting the newspaper sports clippings of her kids in a scrapbook for each of them. She had a couple of visitors come, and when I left I felt an overwhelming sadness.

February 1, 2018

Today was a really good day. She seemed much better. It was nice to have her to myself for a couple of hours. I read her the intro I wrote for this book. She made me do it even though I protested, as I didn't want to cry. I made a promise when she was diagnosed that I would be the strong, stoic friend. She asked me why I didn't want to cry, and I told her I promised myself I wouldn't for her sake. Fran told me sometimes it's good to cry. She said, "I want you to cry, so read it." So, I read it and cried, and it was really, really great. Of course, she smiled while I was crying and reading! We talked about what she wanted regarding the book. We were watching some cooking shows featuring super bowl foods and suddenly she wanted wings. I texted Deanna and she picked up some. Deanna showed up and it was like old times with the three of us. We talked about when we were younger and reminisced about the things we did. We actually got her laughing out loud! Deanna and I felt like we at least got her mind off her disease for a little while. I asked her if there was anything she regretted, or if she could go back, would she change anything? She thought for a moment and said no. Because at the time, she said, she had no way of knowing if it would help. She told me that the things she thought helped control her symptoms the most, such as muscle twitching, were the ketogenic diet, acupuncture, and massage. She said that she wanted to try different treatments so that if she found something that worked, then no one else would have to go through having this disease. When I left that day, I had mixed emotions of happiness and sadness.

February 5, 2018

From Carole's notes:
Dr. Velugubanti prescribed Vitamin B12 1,000 mcg, 1 tablet 1× a day, and Feosol 325 mg, 1 tablet p.o. BID.

February 23, 2018

I stopped by for about forty-five minutes and helped Julie and Terri finish showering and dressing MayFran. She was so tired that all she wanted to do was lay in her bed, and she told me that they decided to call hospice. She has been having trouble swallowing and breathing. I laid in the bed next to her and I told her I thought hospice would be a great help, and that they offer many different services. Went to the basketball game that night and sat next to her, and she told me she's very happy about the book and wants to see what all her friends would write about her. It was a buzzer-beater game and we won by two points! She looks so happy when she is watching her kids play! One of the things that drives me crazy at the games is people will come up and try to talk to her during the game or they pat her on the head. I try to tell them she is trying to watch the game. Everyone means well and wants to say hi. I try to run interference for her so she can enjoy the game.

March 1, 2018

Today was a good day. Came by at lunch to help while Andy was working. Lanette, Terri, and Jen A. were there. Fran looked pretty good. We went over some things for the book. I received a couple of letters and I read them to her, which she loved. Deanna stopped by and then she had a ton of visitors—Maggie, Melody, Robin, and Vanessa. We talked about her hospice visit a little bit and it went well. They are going to stop by several times a week, as it is getting difficult for a lot of the people in our group. We have a bedside commode now. Her neck is very weak, so when we lift her we have to cradle her neck and gently position her to a seated position on the couch. Then we need to put our hands under her armpits to lift her to a standing position. While she is standing, the second lady helps get her undies down and then we set her on the commode. We reverse the process when she is finished. It is almost a delicate dance. She is so tall that our shorter ladies have some difficulty lifting her. After a few hours with people coming in and out, she is absolutely exhausted. Even though it tires her out, she does not like to turn people away when they come to see her.

March 20, 2018

From Carole's notes:
MaryFran is having difficulty swallowing the fifty-plus supplements and Andy wants to stop them. Her mom is worried that she will experience a shock of withdrawal. Her mom has found some Chinese herbs that she thinks will possibly help. Andy and MaryFran agreed to try them, as they are fewer capsules to swallow. She is having trouble eating, not sleeping, upset stomach, and anxiety.

Jun Song is the owner and founder of Herbal ALS Classic Herbal. The capsules are "HerbalMN" and "Balance." There are strict instructions regarding temperature and diet. You have to have lung function tests before and during use. They are from the Netherlands and not FDA approved.

From Carole's notes:
MaryFran feels worse every day. She has increased weakness, shortness of breath, a lot of twitching in her muscles, sweaty palms, heat radiating from her arms and spine. Her mom's observations are increased food intake, though not to what Dr. Song wants. Daily bowel movements, less choking, stable walk with support, voice stronger at times, not as wispy. Amount of urination increased.

The doctor states if she cannot gain weight, she cannot help Fran. Her mom tries to feed her at night, "giving it the old college try." She is down to 90 lbs. (There isn't a date on this entry so I do not know where in March or April this has occurred).

March 28, 2018

Hospice came in for their initial visit. They went over with them what they can do for her care and the services they offer. I was not present for this visit. Apparently, it is not what we thought. They do not provide home care. The nurse just stops in to check on Fran. If Andy gets a nurse, he will have to pay out of pocket. Insurance does not cover the expense. I seriously cannot believe how people can live with this disease and not have a support group. The care is so demanding for one or two family members! The costs are astounding and almost nothing is covered by insurance.

April 11, 2018

Stopped by and Cheryl was cooking. Always smells so good when Cheryl is there! Kim S. was helping out, too. I had to share a couple of stories with Fran. I really feel that the Holy Spirit was moving through me the other night and had to share it with her. She really seemed at peace today, much better than last week. I shared my story with her and she told me she was proud of me. I told her I spoke with a publisher and she was really happy. Deanna and Lisa were coming by later to stay with her for the evening, as Andy was taking Megan to have a college visit at Hillsdale College

April 18, 2018

We had a pretty good visit today. She was watching her beloved Detroit Tigers. Fran was very tired today. Her sister-in-law Nancy was visiting. I had exciting news to go over with her regarding the book! The publisher loved her journals! What's not to love? It was taking a lot of effort for her to speak so I just went over details I needed to discuss going forward. She wanted the proceeds to benefit people in our area who were less fortunate and were diagnosed with ALS. McLaren Northern Michigan had set up a foundation in her name. Also, she wanted athletic scholarships at her beloved St. Francis Xavier School. I told her I would send the book to Oprah, Ellen, and Kelly and Ryan, and wherever else I could so that we could be best-selling authors and find a cure for this disease! This really made her happy. I told her to think about a title. She wants something inspirational but not sappy. Something to draw people in and get them to want to read it. So far, she loved everything I read to her and it really filled me with love. I spoke with Andy and he was really happy we are writing the book. He told me that she is the most positive person he has ever met in his life.

April 22, 2018

Father Denny gave a real great homily today about sacrifice. It was really fitting to our support group for MaryFran. He said sometimes when you are volunteering and sacrificing for others, you don't realize that what you get in return is so much greater than what you are giving. I think our support group realizes that now that we are nearing the end, we have received so much more in return than what we have sacrificed in taking care of MaryFran. Our sacrifices have been time away from our families, which given the circumstances have been totally understood. Many of us have made other "sacrifices"—such as money, made meals, etc.—but he is so right in that what we have received in return is so much greater than what we have given. I think that was how MaryFran always tried to live her life. Think about how good you feel when you give someone something, anything!

April 28, 2018

Carole brought me a box full of stuff to go through. She is trying to help fill in the gaps. She has kept copious notes on some of her alternative treatments. Her love for her daughter is so evident. It is heartbreaking to see how hard she has tried to find a cure, knowing that it is basically a needle in a haystack. MaryFran interjects when she feels something is not relevant to what she wants for her story, and I feel it takes her mind off her illness for a while. As her mom shows me some pictures of her with all her medals and awards, I tease her about being a slacker and I finally get a smile. It gets harder and harder to get that smile, as she is getting so uncomfortable. Chanin comes to help with her hair and brings Brenda from her salon to help with her nails; it really helps MaryFran feel better.

April 30, 2018

We went through some photos with her mom today. Her mom found her early school photos, and I laughed uncontrollably at her expense. The typical 70s and 80s hair and clothes. In some of the photos, she looks like the total jock she was. I think we found the cover photo; it is a great picture of her when she was about three or four years old, and I absolutely love it. Her mouth is open in a laugh that is so MaryFran, and her daughter Megan could be mistaken for her. MaryFran dreamt she had the title of the book. "Jesus Is Stuck in My Gums." I almost fell off my chair laughing. We are always helping pick stuff out of her teeth, and in her dream the communion wafer got stuck. Catholics believe that when the host is consecrated it is the body of Christ. She thought people would definitely pick it up to see what it was about.

She wants me to help Terri with Danny's graduation party. She wants the party to be about him and not about her and ALS. I told her that I will help Terri and we will send out an email to the group and do whatever she wants. I told her she does not need to worry about a thing.

I never thought I would do some of the things I have done for MaryFran. Today I changed her tampon and it wasn't a big deal at all, because I look at her and think, as hard as it is for me it is worse for her to even ask me. My goal until she dies is to make her laugh every time I come visit. I pray every night that she dies in her sleep, so that she does not have to endure this any longer. I have never once heard her complain. Several times she has said that she believes God has given her this diagnosis to spare others from it.

May 1, 2018

Deanna and I spent the afternoon with Fran while Andy worked. Her parents were just getting ready to head back home. We found the bin with a lot of her college and high school memorabilia. It helps keep her occupied, and it is fun to reminisce. We teased her about being a slacker in sports in high school when we found the article about her being inducted into her high school athletic hall of fame. I got her to laugh over some of the photos, which was great because earlier, when I was feeding her a shake, she told me she just wanted everything to be over. I told her that I prayed every night that this would end for her; that actually made her happy and she told me, "Thank you."

May 2, 2018

MaryFran asked me to sit in on the phone conversation with Dr. Song. I really don't agree with what is going on after researching her website, but it is not my journey. Andy has refused and feels that he just does not know what is in the pills and has justifiable concerns. I agree with Andy, but she is begging me with her eyes, so I do. She tells me what to write down to tell her and we wait patiently for the call. MaryFran is only able to swallow four of the five capsules and the doctor is unhappy with that. She is able to follow the instructions regarding clothing, temperature in the home, and trying hard with the food recommendations. The doctor is insistent on the pulmonary function test. That is the only way she can adjust the dosage. I tell her we will try to get a home test but we need to get a doctor's order for one. My personal belief is that she cannot physically do it. I tell the doctor that she is now unable to leave the house but she doesn't seem to understand. She keeps saying how important this test is. She wants her to get another weight. I write everything down for her and tell her husband. He says he will try to locate a home pulmonary function test.

May 3, 2018

Deanna, Cheryl, Lynn, Gina, and I had to have a meeting with MaryFran. Many of our group have now become uncomfortable with her care. She takes it much better than we expected and does not want to make anyone uncomfortable and does not want anyone here who does not want to be. We discussed ways to improve our group and how to help the family better. Deanna did a couple of Bible readings and they just happened to fit the moment. Funny how that happens. She seemed much better today, but Deanna and I noticed that she does not like to be alone. Every time we stepped out of the room for a second, she was constantly calling us back in for little things. I kept telling her that we were here for her and that she has always been a sister to me and I will do whatever I can to help her. Gina and I talked to her about her funeral wishes, and she told us that she hates bugs and does not want to be buried! She is thinking that she might want to donate her body to ALS research and asked me to look into it, as long as it the Catholic Church teachings are okay with it. She would like the care group to have a party and drink margaritas and tell great stories about her after she is gone.

May 4, 2018

I stopped by to see if Andy needed any help; Fran was having a rough morning. It was a torrential downpour and she was insistent on going to acupuncture. Andy did not want to take her out in the rain. MaryFran is pretty stubborn. She agreed to cancel it but then started crying and told me that she really needed it today. She feels that it really relaxes her and helps with some of the symptoms, like the muscle twitches. I told Andy that I will help get her there and I will hold the umbrella over the wheelchair. She looked so desperate that I just could not tell her no. While I was feeding her a breakfast shake, she just broke down crying and told me how upset she was that she was going to miss her kids. I told her that she would be watching them from heaven, just like my dad did for me. I shared with her that after my dad died, for many years I had vivid dreams of him and he was perfectly healthy. My dad never met my children and I told her I had dreams of him with my children doing all the things that he loved to do, like fishing and hunting and holding them after they were born. They were so vivid that when I would wake up it would take me several minutes to remember that he wasn't alive. I told her that I know that God will work through her and her children that way. It really helped to calm her down. I stroked her arms and cried with her. I told her that her kids were going to be fine and that she and Andy have done a great job raising them.

I think she knew this would be the last time she would be able to leave the house. Andy got her in the car and I helped stabilize her neck while he put on the neck brace. It is amazing that she could still walk with assistance. Someone has to hold her from behind and steady her as she takes steps. He loaded the wheelchair and I grabbed the umbrella. I followed him to the office, and while he got her into the wheelchair I held the umbrella. We wheeled her in and got her settled on the table. She asked me to stay and kept telling me thank you. She looked so sad and frail. I stayed until they started the treatment. This was the first time that I felt such an overwhelming feeling of hopelessness and unfairness of this entire situation.

May 10, 2018

Cheryl E. is teaching a few of us MaryFran's bathing routine. She bathed her in bed and is very careful to do one limb at a time, so she won't get cold. She uses a special inflatable sink for washing her hair. There is a special lotion to use on her bony prominences to prevent bed sores. She gets a foaming body cleanser called Medline Remedy that you do not have to rinse off. We need to have a couple of people as backup. Deanna, Lynn, and I offered, as we now feel we must do "whatever it takes." She told us that when she is given her sponge bath, it makes her feel like what Jesus must have felt after he was taken off the cross and was washed. I told her it makes me feel like Holy Thursday, when the priest washes everyone's feet. She says that she just pretends she is royalty, like in *Downton Abby*, and all of us have to dress her. If she doesn't think this way, it really makes her crazy!

May 11, 2018

I spent the morning with MaryFran, planning her funeral. I told her that she has the luxury of knowing that she was going to die soon and the rest of us don't know when we are going to die. We are all going to die and I know how much she likes to be in control, so why not plan it? It was actually quite wonderful. The Catholic Church provides a nice booklet on different readings to choose from. I went through it a couple of days before and highlighted the ones I thought she would like. We discussed some of the readings and actually laughed about a few of them because we thought they were odd choices for a funeral. She asked for my input on one or two and I think we did a pretty good job reflecting her in the choices. We chose her favorite songs and picked out who she wanted to read and sing. Her son does readings at church and she would really like for him to participate, but I told her although he is a good reader I was worried that he might not be able to hold it together. We thought she should have a backup, just in case. She asked me, as I also do readings at church, and I honestly told her I didn't think I could hold it together. She looked at me and she said, "I know you will be able to do it." She also wanted her sister to read, hoping she would be able to do it. If not, we have a backup for her. Her niece is an amazing singer, as is one of our girlfriends, and we are going to ask them to sing. It was very important to her that I tell our priest that they not say that she fought ALS. She said it absolutely drives her crazy. We joked that I would tell them that if they say that at the funeral, she will come back and haunt them! She also wanted to include a special intention for all of the friends and their families who helped take care of her throughout her illness. She made me promise that I would make sure there would be a special Frantabulous Friends memorial party, where we would drink margaritas (her favorite) and tell stories about her and celebrate her life in a positive way. I told her if margaritas were involved, I would absolutely make sure it would happen!

May 18, 2018

Stopped by today to go over a few things for the "celebration of life." I had met with Father Denny the day before and he wanted me to make sure I followed up on a couple of things. Danny came home, and we went up to talk with his mom. She asked him to read at her celebration of life. He asked her if she really wanted him to. She said yes. Danny is a very accomplished reader at our church. I talked to him afterward and told him that his mom asked me to be the backup, if he was too upset the day of the funeral. I told him that we would wait right up to the last minute. He said okay, but he really didn't want to let his mom down. She did not look good today. Her breathing is getting worse and so is her speech. She is developing sores on her ears from lying on them and not being able to turn her head. She is not comfortable sitting up, so she lays down the whole day. We have to be very careful now, so she does not get bedsores.

May 30, 2018

I came by for a little bit to help Terri get ready for Danny's graduation party. MaryFran just seems increasingly frail every time I come. Her breathing is much more, shallow. I fed her a little bit; I still can't believe she's able to eat. This is the first time that I really had to decipher what she was trying to say to me. I can see she's trying to control everything for the graduation party even though she knows she has very little control over anything, and it is so hard on her. Deanna is setting up her laptop so that we can use FaceTime for her to see what's going on at the party, as she just does not feel she can be physically present.

May 31, 2018

I picked up the flower arrangements for the party and headed over to help set up. Deanna and I did a run through with FaceTime again so that MaryFran could stay in her bed and watch. She did not want to have a lot of visitors up in her room and wanted the party to be about Danny. It was working out pretty well; people were saying hi to her via the phone. We had a few stragglers trying to sneak up, and we explained to them that it was too overwhelming for her. There were a couple of people who chose not to listen, and it really stressed her out. They really don't understand how claustrophobic she gets.

They had a really great turn out for the party; overall, I think everything went really well.

June 1, 2018

I did not stop by, but I heard from another friend that MaryFran had a really rough day and the party took a lot out of her. I just wish sometimes that there was more that we could do to help ease her transition. I know she would really like to attend the graduation ceremony on Sunday, but I just don't know how she's going to do it because she cannot even sit up anymore. Deanna talked to the school and they said they would disable the block on FaceTime so that the family could possibly set that up for her, so she can watch it live from her bedroom.

June 3, 2018

Graduation day for Danny! MaryFran was not able to attend. Terri stayed home with her while the family attended the baccalaureate mass and graduation ceremony. Megan took videos with her phone, so she could share them with her mom.

June 4, 2018

My life is consumed by MaryFran now. As the group-care coordinator, not a day goes by without texts, calls, or emails about Fran. At this point we are all praying for her to die peacefully. It has taken a toll on everyone. Terri and I decided to tour Hiland Cottage, so we can see for ourselves what they offer, and we needed to meet with the funeral director to finalize the details, to make an easier transition for the kids. MaryFran told Terri she does not want to die at home. I think this is for the best, and so does just about everyone else. Her care is too much for our group now. She needs skilled nursing that most of us are unable to provide.

June 5, 2018

The meeting with the funeral director went well. He gave us some great advice. He told us that one thing families share with him is they wished they had put their family member in Hiland Cottage sooner. (I encourage anyone with a terminal illness to tour this facility or any facility in your area that is similar, before it is too late.) It may not be what you choose, but at least you will have options. You are also familiar with it before it becomes time to decide.

June 10, 2018

Lisa, Deanna, and I are on this week. All three of us are nervous because her care is getting so difficult. Deanna has decided that she no longer wants to feed her anymore because last week Fran almost choked on her. School is now out so Lisa is available during the day, which is great. Natalie came down for a quick visit. I think mostly to say good-bye because; we all know the end is near. She's only staying 'til the afternoon. Deanna is going on vacation on Friday, so Lisa and I decided we will stop by the house on Monday morning at 10 a.m. to see what Andy needs for the rest of the week.

June 11, 2018

We stopped by to check in with Andy and he assures us he is okay, except for Tuesday, when he works. Lisa will come back after Natalie leaves so that Andy can run some errands with Danny. He needs a vehicle for college. I stay for a little bit with Natalie to show her some of the book. I don't want to intrude on her time with Fran, as she lives downstate, so I offered to email her what I have. I explained to her that I have shown MaryFran about 95 percent of the book. I have not shared all of my journals, as I am not sure if they will be included. She is overcome with emotion and is so thankful for our support group. I tell Fran I love her and will stop by tomorrow. She tells me she loves me more and gives me a smile. I give her a kiss on the forehead.

Lisa and I were supposed to come early and bathe her, but Jen and Terri let us know that they will come at 10 and do it. Lisa will come at 12:30 and then I will come shortly after. I have a meeting in the evening and Deanna will come in the afternoon.

June 12, 2018

We had a change in plans. Terri decided she's going to stay the whole day. She texted me in the morning that Fran is having a rough day and told Deanna and me that we can have a day off. Frankly, I am relieved, as I have a lot going on in my personal life, and so does Deanna, as she is packing for her trip. Every day, I am answering texts and emails from the group. I also work for my husband, but luckily, I can do a lot on my trusty iPad.

Lisa called me that evening and told me that it was very rough. She wished that Deanna and I could have been there to help out, but Fran did not want any other visitors. Lisa cooked and ran errands while Terri took care of Fran. Unfortunately, Fran started to become incontinent and was very upset.

Terri texted me and asked if I could come at 11 the next day so that Andy could run to the grocery store. I told her absolutely.

June 13, 2018

I spoke with Katie this morning. Her week is coming up, and she is nervous about what to expect. I told her that, unfortunately, it's a day-by-day thing. She is still eating through a straw. It takes great effort for her to speak—it's barely a whisper and difficult to understand. I told her to pray for a bed to open up.

I got a text from Andy at 9:12 a.m. that a bed opened up. He said Fran is willing to give it a try.

I am so relieved for her, her family, and for our group. He asked if I could still come at 11. I told him I would do whatever he needed me to do today to help. I have mixed emotions. I am sad but relieved. I let Deanna and Lisa know.

I got there a little before 11. I am nervous; not sure what to expect. Terri is with Fran and I go over to say hi. We are waiting to hear what time the transport is coming. I try to stay out of the way but available. Andy comes back with groceries, and the kids and I help put them away. It is agony waiting. Terri and I prepare some food and try to keep things "normal." I talk to the kids about how great the cottage is; they are ready for her to go. They need to have their house back and to have a sense of normalcy. Meg tells us about coaching volleyball camp and Danny is excited about the upcoming college orientation. I feel like an intruder but feel so very honored to be included. I realize at this moment that as horrible as losing MaryFran is, they will be okay. Andy is a great dad and Terri is a wonderful aunt. I sit with Fran for a little bit and give her some water. She asks Terri and I to get a few more things to bring with her. She has a beautiful Jesus painting she wants, and I run to grab it. Transport gets there around 12:30. Being a small town, we of course know Cal, one of the EMTs. As they load her onto the stretcher, it is everything I can do not to breakdown. I know this is the last time she will be home and is now truly headed toward her death. I cannot lose it in front of her kids. They are doing surprisingly okay. True to form, as they wheel her by us she gives a big smile. She is still directing us what to do and Andy tells her, "Franny, you are still running the show." The kids follow Andy in the ambulance. Terri, Craig, and I clean up all of the medical detritus so that when the kids come back it is not such a reminder. Andy texts that a few more things are needed, and we will take turns running them over.

When the kids get back they are happy with how nice the cottage is. They talk about spending the night there and are happy she will be cared for. I tell them that I am putting out the family time signs and they can leave them for as long as they like. They are so happy and relieved.

Danny tells me, "Thank you so much." I tell him everyone needs to knock on the door now.

I run over a few things she needed and some of the flower arrangements. Just as I get there the hospice doctor shows up. I stop, unsure whether I should leave or stay. Nobody looks at me or asks me to leave, so I just go about putting things away. Fran's ALS presents differently than typical ALS, if there is a typical presentation. She can still move her legs a little bit but her whole upper body is basically useless. The doctor comments on this. She also goes over her requests regarding feeding tube, vent, and DNR. Fran does not want any of this except the DNR. By this time, I decide to sit on the couch in the sunroom, out of the way but nearby if they need me.

Dr. Maggie and Andy come over and sit with me. Andy introduces me; Maggie knows my husband—small town! I explain to her about Frantabulous Friends. She cannot believe the size of our group and how we have cared for her. She lays down the "rules" of Hiland Cottage for me to email to the group. She asks that we let the nurses take over her care, but we let them know Fran's preferences. I go over with Andy and Fran what they would like in the email and she is more worried about Danny's birthday, which is tomorrow. I give her a kiss good-bye. I tell her I love you! She whispers I love you more! I leave around 4 and I am exhausted. I send the email and I am inundated with texts and emails. It's all good. I want to reassure everyone; I want to do what I can for their family. My husband and son have been wonderful and patient through all of this.

June 15, 2018

I stop briefly. She can barely whisper. She has so many visitors. She loves the visitors, but she is so tired. Maggie found a way on Google forms for people to sign up for an hour at a time to sit and visit. We will try this so someone is with her from 10 a.m.–8 p.m., then Andy can have a break. People can still stop in if they want. It is a steady stream of visitors. Andy stays the night every night with her. He truly is an amazing husband.

June 18, 2018

My husband and I go visit Fran for a few minutes. He hasn't had a chance to see her in a long time. She is tired and restless, so we don't stay long.

June 19, 2018

I have a migraine and debate all morning about going. I feel like something is pulling me to go see her, so I go and there are a lot of visitors. I talk to Andy for a few minutes to see if I need to send out anything new in an email, and he tells me no. I don't want to intrude on other's time with her, as I feel blessed to have had a lot of special moments with her, so I just wave hi and tell Andy to tell her I love her and that I will see her when I get back from a short trip to Mackinac Island.

June 20, 2018

Andy texted me at 8:20 a.m. MaryFran passed away at 8 a.m. The kids and Andy were with her and she went peacefully. I am sad, yet happy she is now with Jesus. I will miss who she was before her diagnosis. I am glad she is no longer suffering, though she never complained. ALS has changed me and made me a better person, but I will forever hate this disease. Her ALS journey is over.

June 25, 2018

Today is her visitation and vigil. I spent the last couple of days fielding texts, emails, Facebook messages from people wanting to know the dates and times of the visitation and celebration. I hope and pray everything will be as she wished. Natalie and Melody worked on the photo boards. Deanna is on vacation and is working on a video that she sends to me at about three o'clock. I email it to Deacon Paul and he is able to burn a

DVD so that we can play it on the TVs in the gathering space. I watch it in my car and can't help but cry and smile at the same time.

The photos are absolutely stunning. They are blown up and on easels, all through the gathering space. The DVD is streaming, and it is perfect. The flowers are beautiful in her favorite colors. St. Francis Xavier Church is a very large church and Andy is at the front, greeting people; the line is out the door. It stays that way until the start of the vigil. They have her ashes in a wooden box engraved with her name, surrounded by flowers with her wedding portrait, and it is breathtaking. I thought that I could handle it, and my breath catches in my throat. My husband senses my distress and grabs my hand, and I say to him, "I can't look it at it. It's too much for me." He gently leads me away, so I can compose myself. We talk with our friends until the vigil starts.

The readings are beautiful and Deacon Paul's eulogy wonderfully sums up MaryFran. He spent a lot of time with her and really got to know her. Andy starts with the speeches. I do not know how he is able to give such a loving tribute. He breaks down several times but gives the most wonderful, loving, heartfelt speech. The love he has for Fran is so evident that I think every woman in attendance is jealous of her! All men could take a lesson from the husband handbook of Andy. Though I am sure he would readily admit all the mistakes he made through their marriage, there is no doubt that Fran was the love of his life. Her parents and sister give touching tributes. My husband is elbowing telling me that I need to get up and talk on behalf of the care group. I tell him that I have not prepared anything and I don't think I can do it. Those that know me, I am never at a loss for words! Fred tells me I have to. Danny gets up and speaks and it is heartbreaking, yet a wonderful tribute to his mother and the relationship they had. Megan is next and she breaks the ice with a touching and hilarious speech. With her courage and lightening of the mood, I now know I can do it. I make it through and think I do a decent job and hope it comes off as I want. Several more people speak and we finally close. It is a loving tribute to a woman that touched many people.

I get home, and to unwind I decide to play a few games of words with friends against the computer. I am shocked when the first computer person I play is named Franni. Call me crazy but I do not believe this is a coincidence.

June 26, 2018

Today is the day of the celebration of life. Surprisingly, I am not nervous. I know I've done everything she wished. I just hope everything goes as planned. It is in God's hands now. My son John wanted to be an altar server for the service. I know he will do a great job. The family is very close with two priests, and Father Denny will be the main celebrant with Father Mathew as the co-celebrant. I am very surprised to see Bishop Lynch and Father Brad. I almost laughed out loud and thought only MaryFran would be able to get a bishop, three priests, a seminarian, and a deacon to preside over her service! Her niece Dana sings as a soloist and is amazing. Everything is perfect and exactly as we discussed—from music, readings, and Father's eulogy is simply amazing. She would have loved it. I felt like there was an aura shining through the church that day, an indescribable light shining onto the altar.

We head over for the luncheon and I hope we can pull off the margarita toast as planned. We gather the ladies from the group in the parking lot and a few others join us. Marie has a five-gallon cooler and Julie brought cups and ice. We were hoping to grab Andy but didn't want to take him away from his family. But wouldn't you know, I am pretty sure Fran was watching over us because just as we were almost ready, I see Andy walking across the lot and I wave him over. He asks me, "What are you guys up to?" I tell him MaryFran made me promise to do a margarita toast at the luncheon. He throws his head back and laughs and says to me she would have loved this. We raise our glasses and I give a short but sweet toast and take a sip of our delicious margaritas. It made everything perfect. We decided we needed a group photo with Andy in the center to commemorate the occasion. The lunch is wonderful. Marie wrote a song and some of the ladies in the group sing it at the end of the luncheon.

Marie is famous for her little ditties. My son summed it up best. He told me, "Mom, I know you helped plan this, but I have served a lot of funerals and this was the most beautiful funeral I have ever served."

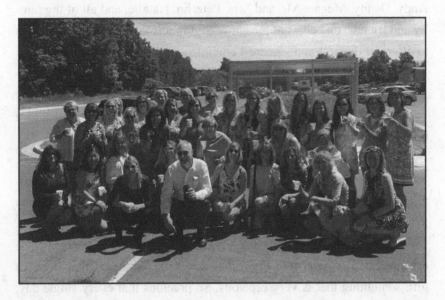

June 29, 2018

I stopped by at the cemetery today. I needed a couple of days to grieve. I tell MaryFran, "I hope you loved everything because I think everything was perfect. I miss you, but I am forever grateful I had this time as your friend."

I have included Deacon Paul's eulogy and Father Denny's homily. I feel that in this day and age of discord, they are so beautiful that they need to be shared.

Deacon Paul's Eulogy

MaryFran Kolp Vigil, June 25, 2018
First reading: Revelation 14:13: "Blessed are the Dead for their Good Deeds go with Them."

Psalm 27: "The Lord is My Light and Salvation."
Gospel: Matthew 11:25–30: "Come to Me and I will Give You Rest."

Andy, Danny, Megan, Mr. and Mrs. Peterlin, Natalie, and all of the family and friends, on behalf of the entire St. Francis faith community, I wish to offer our deepest and sincerest condolences on the loss of MaryFran.

You all are bearing some heavy crosses now.

Andy, you lost your love.

Danny and Megan, it is really hard to lose your mother. It leaves a hole in your heat that really never can be completely healed.

Mr. and Mrs. Peterlin, I am so sorry. No parent should bury their child.

Natalie, next to parents, siblings are with you from almost the beginning of your life. The grief you are experiencing right now is hard for us to comprehend.

Even though MaryFran's death was expected and she bore the heaviest cross, it is events like these that are stark reminders that life is a gift, something that is very precious. So precious that every single day, and every relationship we have, is a gift that should never be taken for granted.

When we lose a beloved wife, mother, daughter, sister, aunt, and friend, we are at a loss to make sense on an aspect of life that seems impossible to understand.

The gospel passage from Matthew just proclaimed is a comforting one. And one we have probably heard many times before. In fact, it is the first reading of choice for the sacrament of the anointing of the sick.

Yet our culture is so far removed from Jesus' time, we miss some of its meaning and richness.

Jesus says, "Take my yoke upon you and learn from me, for I am meek and humble of heart. And you will find rest for yourselves. For my yoke is easy, and my burden light."

How can a yoke be easy? The very fact a yoke is being used means that the pull will be a tough one. How can you find rest by taking on a yoke?

And how can a burden be light? If a burden were light, it wouldn't be a burden.

Yokes are used to pair up oxen, to distribute the weight and make their load easier to pull and to make it more comfortable. Yokes are typically custom made for a specific pair of oxen. Usually, the pair is made up of oxen that are of unequal size and strength. Those oxen bear the same burden together, and because of that yoke it makes the load easier for both.

When life is at its darkest, we may not realize it, but it is exactly when God is closest to us. When there are no answers, yet Jesus is still at our side. He is there, whether we know it or not, bearing our burden right along with us and helping us to shoulder our yoke. He is the Big Ox pulling more than his share for the team.

He also uses us to help others bear and lighten their burden.

All you ladies who made up the crew that seemed to be a constant presence at Andy and MaryFran's home, what you did was incredible. The atmosphere at the house on visits was always welcoming, warm, upbeat, and cheerful.

When MaryFran couldn't use her arms, you became her hands. When she could no longer care for herself, you cared for her. The weaker she became, the stronger you became, and in turn made her strong. You made her yoke easy, and the tremendous burden she had to bear, light.

MaryFran is truly blessed to have all of you.

God was right there with MaryFran, and supported her and inspired all of you to be His instruments, so that through you He brought consolation, strength, and courage to MaryFran so that she could face all the challenges that came her way.

MaryFran is a very special person.

When I visited MaryFran, more often than not, I felt she ministered to me more than I ministered to her.

I will never forget her.

There is a fifth-century Latin hymn that starts with this line…

Ubi caritas est amor, Deus ibi est. Where charity and love are, there God is.

The opening song we just sang is based on that hymn.

Charity is here,
caring loving people are here,
and God is right here now.

Everyone's presence here says more than any words can. We are all grieving in our own way and are here to support each other.

Danny and Megan, I have one more insight on the yoke and Big Ox for you. Up to now, MaryFran, along with Andy, was your Big Ox. I know she loved you very much. She spoke of you often, was very proud of you, and deeply cared for you both.

I think she would tell you that now is the time to take over her part of being the Big Ox for your family now, your future families, and all the people you will have the opportunity to share your lives with and touch. Just look around here and see all the hearts she touched, and there are many more besides. Remember all the things MaryFran did for you and others.

We are all truly blessed to have had MaryFran touch our lives.

Our Lord said, "I am the resurrection and the life. If anyone believes in me, even though he dies, yet he will live."

You see, the whole point of our faith is that when we are met with this fear of darkness and death, we are not ashamed to call out. Because the whole point of believing is the conviction that there is someone there who will answer. And that someone is God.

Godspeed, MaryFran.

Danny Kolp Memorial Speech to his Mother

I usually have a well-prepared speech that she helps me with every time. I remember she told me after we beat TC Central—at TC Central my senior year in basketball—to not regret anything, and so that's why I am up here. I remember she told me, quote, "Every book has a beginning and an end, and that's why we live each day to the fullest." I think that speaks really well for itself. I was with my aunt Nat a couple of days ago when she came in, and I remember her talking about why we live, and although my mom's only fifty and would be fifty-one this July 3, it's as though she has lived 150 years. She was a people person, and being her son, I wanted to be a people person. I did everything I could to be with my mom every day. I know we don't always have the best days, but that is what builds character. My mom definitely had character. From AU tournaments, to traveling the country, going to Vegas, Los Angeles, New York City, Boston, Atlanta, I've been all over the country; there's no other place I'd rather grow up than in Petoskey. I think that has a lot to do with you guys. The community was something special for her. She was someone who lived by example. She didn't have to say the words for you to understand it; she simply lived it. I remember her telling me that she was happy that she had to go through it so that no one else had to. That was the hardest thing for me to understand. I have been telling a lot of you people whom I have said hi to that she would not want us to be sad but to be happy, and I don't think that is any more, true, than today. She has affected so many people, and in so many different ways. There is not a day that won't go by that I won't think about her. I remember as she got sicker, for my grad party it was May 28th, and probably for a month before that, she should've been in the hospital bed. She didn't want other people to see her like that. I think that shows the strength she had. She was the strongest person I ever met. And I know she would want to say thank you to everyone. Going through hard things in life builds character. Although I just turned nineteen, that is something I will always remember. Frantabulous. So, be as selfless as she was and make this world a better place.

My Completely Unplanned, Heartfelt Speech

I want to thank Megan because I didn't think I would be able to come up here. For those of you who don't know me, I am Kim Wroblewski, and I am the head of the care group. I was appointed by MaryFran to be the head of the care group. Those of you who don't know, a lot of the time you don't get a say in these things. We met twenty-one years ago and she kind of guides you, and as Natalie said, once you meet her that's pretty much it. We found that we had a lot of similar interests and we parented the same and we had similar ideals in raising our kids. You know, through her diagnosis, I just found it really changed me for the better, even though we went through a lot. I never imagined I could grow as a person. But the one thing I won't miss before the texting and emails was my call, "Hey, Kim. It's Fran. Hey, you want to go to this?" or "Hey, the school needs this. We got to go volunteer. I signed you up."

I would go, "Ugh, what are we going to do now?"

"Come on. We're going to go do this! We volunteered for the medical alliance, we were co-presidents of that." We volunteered for the school and church.

I volunteered so much with her, and she's right, you know? I always felt better. We always did so much together, and up until the end it was always, "Kim, come over here. Okay, this is what I want you to put in the email. Don't forget this. Kim don't forget this."

And I would go, "I got it, Fran. I got it. I know what you want me to say."

"It's Danny's birthday, Kim. Don't forget to put in the email it's Danny's birthday."

"I got it, Fran. Don't worry about it."

But I want to say to this care group, all these women, a lot of them I knew a bit, but we became such a family. I think we're forever bonded because of her. We were maybe a little friendly, but for the rest of our lives we are in it. And you three, if you think that you are rid of us? Because your mom made me promise, you're not going to forget about them, right? You're still going to bring the meals? Promise me you're not going to forget? I told her we're going to take care of them.

Andy told me, "Kim, you know I do know how to cook, right?"

I am like, "Andy, please just let me do this. You know how she is. You can't say no."

And for those of you who don't know, Fran had asked me—or told me—that I was going to help her write a book about her journey. We have probably completed about 90 percent of it. When she talked to me about it, I was like, "I really don't know if I can handle that." But it has been a wonderful journey to do this with her, and even though we didn't find a cure she felt it was so important to put out there what she went through so that other people, if they got dealt this horrible diagnosis, they could at least go somewhere, that they could find a book where your faith is so strong. She wanted to be positive in facing such a horrible diagnosis and show where people come together and show how your faith could help you. Show all her treatments and everything that she tried. I asked her one day if there was anything that she would've changed or done differently.

She said, "No, because how would I know if something would work or not? If something would've worked, I could save somebody else from having to go through this, and maybe somebody could get a care group or maybe they could find friends like I have, and it would make a difference in someone else's life and they wouldn't have to go through this."

I love her for that. I will miss those phone calls, but nobody else can call me and ask me to do this again because she was special. Everyone keeps telling me that they can't believe I did this for her, but I know she would've done the same thing for me in a minute. Just remember, you two (pointing to Danny and Megan) you are not rid of us yet.

Father Dennis Stilwell's Eulogy

I am very happy this morning to welcome Bishop Lynch, and Father Matthew has returned. On behalf of all of us here, I would like to extend our condolences to you, Andy, Danny, and Megan, on the loss of your beautiful wife and mother.

We are here this morning to celebrate something that's very, very important for all of us, and what we're celebrating, it is that love never dies. Love never dies. That was what St. Paul said. He said everything passes away. But not love. Love is eternal. Jesus said whoever abides in love, abides in God, and I don't think that there could ever be anything more consoling to us that we are believers, than that promise that love never dies.

Well, MaryFran wanted her funeral to be a celebration of life and love. No black. Do you see any black up here? No black. She wanted colors so we're wearing colors. We can celebrate life and love as MaryFran requested. Because we know that MaryFran abided in love, therefore she abided in God who is eternal. And now MaryFran is eternal. She chose the readings; she chose everything—music—and everything that she chose filled with hope and promise and joy. Just as she was filled with all of that.

I think in my forty-seven years of presiding over funerals, I have never heard or saw or experienced what I did in the Kolp home during these past months. A virtual army of volunteers coming forward out of sheer love for MaryFran. Around the clock, giving MaryFran so much that she needed in terms of love and caring and so on, but they were not the only ones who were doing the loving and giving. I think MaryFran, maybe was doing consoling and comforting as much as she was being consoled and comforted.

But also, in the way that she chose not to die but to live until her last breath, her attitude was filled with a really profound gratitude for life that have been given her, and that life that she was able to share with Andy and Danny and Megan, and all of us. I mean that's a lot of loving and caring life to share with all of us, so many of us. MaryFran's home was and always had been home wherein love was both given and received. A home where everybody is welcome, and you can feel it, feel something special in that home. I don't know if you were all able to identify it yourself, but what you felt was that God abided in the Kolp home. It affected everybody who visited that home. So, what we experience at the Kolp home, I believe, was an authentic experience of the Kingdom of God. Because the Kingdom of God is all about real love and real love is all about what Christ said when he said, "Father, I pray that they will love each other as you and I love each other." The commitment and the willingness to do whatever it took, whatever sacrifices were necessary, in order to be the family that was needed to be with all those friendships, all those people coming together. You know, it is something marvelous to behold when we see human beings truly being human and the way that God designed us to be, and that is when we care for each other, giving and receiving love. Who was it that said that when life is given and received, one's life is successful? Human beings need love. We not only give what we have, but we give who and what we are, and that was so obvious in the Kolp home. So, this whole dynamic was present in the Kolp home, and when we enter into the dynamic, it affects us and something within us changes.

I love the Chinese proverb that says a bit of fragrance always clings to the hand that gives you roses. MaryFran gave out an awful lot of roses and fragrance has clung to all of us. There's nothing more beautiful than human beings just being human the way God created us to be. It's amazing how often we forget that. There's a wonderful law of nature that the things we crave most in life, freedom and peace of mind, are always attained by giving them to someone else. Look back on the most for filling happy moments of your life and you'll be able to connect the dots because that's when you gave of yourself sacrificially for all the right reasons without the holding back. That makes life so good. I think this seems to be a summary of MaryFran's life. I know that last night at the wake, a number of you shared some memories and experiences of how

MaryFran touched your life. So, I would like to give him my own memory of MaryFran. I think the one that sticks out the most. You know, shortly after I got here, I tried to get organized an annual dinner auction that would raise a lot of money for our school. Because schools need a lot of money and so on, gradually, over time, it came to be on one of those occasions, MaryFran had directed and guided our parish through that whole dynamic and we had a very successful dinner auction. But then things began to fall apart. I mean they really just completely fell apart. I knew that we were going to be in a lot of trouble if we didn't have the fund-raiser, so I called MaryFran and she knew what was going on. I asked her if she would take charge, and then we would organize this and give it new life—and she said, "Absolutely! Don't worry about it!" I was scared to death that I would have to beg her. But she said, "Absolutely! Don't worry about it at all. It will be done."

So now what? Where do all of us go from here? So many of us were in the Kolp home, so many of us were there hour after hour, day after day, week after week, giving of our time and of ourselves to administer to MaryFran. So now all of that's over. So now what? No doubt we are relieved, and at peace that her suffering is over. I think not so much that her suffering is over but because we know where she is. Love never dies. Everything else does, but not love. We know that on this earth God abided in her, and she in God. And there's every reason to believe that that is not changed. She abides in God and God in her, and she continues to abide in all of us. You know, as time passes memories fade. It's the natural way of things, but there are some people, some special people, who touch us on such a level that it takes a very long time for their memory to fade. Sometimes it never does. Because we can always recall the way that someone had touched us, the way it made a difference in us and perhaps caused change to take place in us. What an incredible gift that is. There is no better gift to give to another than the gift of self. Selfless love is when God gives Himself to us. So, you know, we still have own life span to live, however long. Perhaps MaryFran has taught us how to walk through this life with grace, with beauty, with hope, and with love. We're

celebrating a life well lived, a life that has touched us all, and how grateful we are and that our hearts are filled with joy and how good God is.

◆◆◆◆◆

In August, I invited the ladies from the Frantabulous Friends group
to my home for a little lunch and margaritas. I had to fulfill my last promise to MaryFran. I wanted to do something special and finally came up
with an idea that I had hoped would be meaningful and in the spirit of
"MaryFran." Not everyone could come, but I think I had at least fif-
teen people show up. I waited 'til I felt was the right time and I handed
out the packages and margaritas and told them they could open them.
Inside was either a group photo from our margarita toast at MaryFran's
funeral—or if they couldn't attend the funeral, I found a photo of them
with MaryFran to give them. I also included a Hershey bar. I told them
about MaryFran's Hershey bar story, which she told all of the teams she
coached, and how we were MaryFran's team, but now that she is gone
our team is broken. But just because she is gone it doesn't mean that we
won't forever share a bond. They all wanted to make sure they could eat
the Hershey bar, and I laughed and said absolutely! It ended up being a
beautiful day and we had a great time!

PART 4

Part 4

MaryFran asked friends to write letters to her about how they met and how her diagnosis changed their lives in a positive way. It turned into a beautiful exercise in dealing with grief, but also showing how something horrible can help people make changes in their lives. They were given the choice to come and read them to her personally, or if they did not feel they could, I was given the honor of reading them to her. This became one of our favorite things to do. It helped us go down memory lane, which is always fun, but more importantly, you learn how small acts of kindness over the course of your life truly affect others. I wanted to include them in the book, not to make her a martyr, but to show how even though everyone is imperfect, you never know how you can make a difference in someone's life. I love that she got to know before she passed that she truly affected others' lives.

Ode to MaryFran
by Kristin J.

I met MaryFran when I started working here at St. Francis over ten years ago. I don't remember the exact moment, but I do remember being jealous of Mrs. Mac because she got to have Danny in her class and I didn't. You always want the kids with the good parents. It just makes the year a lot smoother. MaryFran was one of those parents you wanted to have.

I did get to teach Megan, though. I had her in fourth grade but only for a half of a day due to the schedule Molly McCarthy and I ran. Megan was a joy and having MaryFran around was wonderful. She was a breath of fresh air. The moment that stuck out the most that year was when we went on our Lansing trip. It was my first time teaching fourth grade, which meant it was my first time taking a class to Lansing. Molly's daughter got very sick the day that we were heading down and wasn't able to go, sticking me with the trip by myself. Immediate panic. MaryFran came over, told me that we have this, and that it was going to be awesome. And it was. She took the reins, showed me where to be and what to do, and ultimately saved the day.

MaryFran was always the mom and woman around school you wanted to be. Always upbeat, the "cool" mom, her kids loved her and was okay with having her around, the friend you always wanted to have. To me she was the cool older kid at school you would hope notice you. She always noticed. She made me feel welcome, equal, and a friend even though I felt like the dorky little sister.

I look up to her still. The faith that she and Andy have instilled in her children is amazing. I admire Danny for reading and involving himself in church. Not many high school seniors make the time for their faith. I look at my three boys and hope they turn out like him. Every time we see him, I make a point to mention his name: "Look, there's Danny Kolp doing the first reading." "There is Megan, his sister; she was a student of mine." "Brock, look, Danny is at SST, too, trying to improve his game." If my boys turn out like Danny, I will be blessed beyond words.

MaryFran being sick has made me look at my life differently. I want to enjoy everything and experience it now before it may be too late. I want to be friends with the Lord and welcome whatever comes to be whenever it does. And I want to live my life including everyone, being friendly to everyone, and being happy with what I have. MaryFran has made me a better person and impacted me more than I know. Thank you, MaryFran.

Of course, I knew who you were before I had Danny in fourth grade. Who didn't know you? You, MaryFran, are a legend at St. Francis. Larger than life, helper to all, kind, giving, considerate, caring. To say that I was excited to have you as a parent in my class would be a huge understatement.

I can't remember how many kids were in that class, but I think it was around twenty...and if memory serves, only six of them were girls. That was a boy-heavy class. And what a group of personalities we had! You know...every class has its share of bright kids, struggling kids, button pushers, helpers, talkers, etc. This comes with the territory. Every teacher knows this. You roll with the punches, change things up, do what you need to do to make a difference in the lives of each and every child. But it's the parents who can make or break a year for the teacher.

You were a breath of fresh air for me. You were real. I could talk with you, laugh, joke. I could tell you if Danny was say, caught swearing (ha-ha) or talking too much, or being a wonderful, loving kid. He, of course, was all of that and more. I have loved that boy for the past nine years. And I get tears in my eyes every time I see him as a reader at mass, or he wraps me in a bear hug, or he tells me that his career as a reader at mass started in my classroom. Oh, the pride I feel when I watch that boy.

Now here is the kicker...I got to have you as a parent two years in a row! Do you know how exciting that is for a teacher? I was elated to know that Megan was coming up the next year and that I would get to spend a second year with you. Now Megan's class...that was a gem of a class. Man, I loved those kids. I have never had a group of kids so driven to succeed. That class was one for the record books for me. And Meg... bright, kind, loving...just like her mama. You must be so proud. Meg was such an amazing young lady. I get the chance to see her every now and then and I always get a hug, and I always get a smile, and it just warms my heart. She is such a poised, beautiful young woman. I'm so proud to have had a small part in her development.

I remember riding with you in Danny's year to Lansing. So much fun. I remember my mom (also known as Mrs. Crabtree) putting Andy in the dunce seat at the One Room School. She told him to look at Thomas Jefferson's rules and to memorize one. Then she asked him what he learned. He said something like, "Always put off until tomorrow what you should do today." That got a huge laugh. The next year, she put him back in and told him he better learn the saying right this time. He was such a great sport.

Even after your kids moved on from fourth grade, you continued to be one of my strongest supporters, and I have always appreciated that. Teaching is not for the weak. We get beat up quite regularly. If it wasn't for parents like you, I know I would not have made it to this point in my career. You have always been a bright, shining star for me. For that, I thank you.

I'm not going to lie...your diagnosis threw me for a loop. I thought, How, could this be? How is it even possible? I felt lost. I wanted to help. I didn't know if I could. I'm a crier...always have been, always will be. I could never fit in with British society, stiff upper lip and all that. I cry all the time. I knew that wasn't what you needed. I was thrilled to be able to make a quilt for you with my class. I loved putting together a poetry anthology for you. I threw my heart into that project...knowing that it was one small thing that I could do. I knew people were making meals, and driving to appointments, but those tasks were just not in the cards for me. I didn't own a car. I wish I could have done more. I hope you know you have been in my heart and my mind since the minute I heard about the diagnosis.

Your diagnosis has helped me look at the world through different lenses. I appreciate more. I care more. I take nothing and nobody for granted. It helped me realize what a gift life and health are.

I love you, MaryFran, and I love your family. I am sending this story wrapped up in every ounce of care and compassion that I have inside of me.

—Molly M.

I have two stories to share about Fran. The first I will entitle "You Reap What You Sow." I can't remember exactly where or when Fran and I first met, but I know it was when our boys were in preschool at St. Francis. What I do recall is how incredibly welcoming and friendly she was. If there was a new family in school, you could bet that Fran was going to invite the children over for a playdate, and she was for sure going to invite the mother out for a "girls' night out." She made sure that no one was left out. She gave new meaning to the phrase "no child left behind"! Her positive energy was contagious. Little did she know that all of the friendships that she formed when the kids were growing up would be invaluable after she was diagnosed with ALS. Fran cultivated an amazing group of both women and men who were more than willing to reach out and help in any way possible. Lesson learned...you reap what you sow.

My second story is called "Kindred Spirits?" On July 3, 2014, my family went to visit my parents in the eastern Upper Peninsula. My dad had recently been diagnosed with recurrent prostate cancer. I arrived at my parents' home, took one look at my dad in his rocking chair, and dropped to my knees in tears. Dad had a myriad of issues going on, and they had taken a toll on him. Later that day, on the eve of July 3, I received the text that Fran had been officially diagnosed with ALS. I knew very little about ALS, so I spent some time with Google. Very quickly, I learned that one of my dearest friends was facing the fight of her life. That month, my mom, sister, and I went on a road trip with Dad to Mayo Clinic. Dad came home from Mayo with a newfound energy to fight his own battle. For both Fran and my dad, the years to follow were consumed with countless doctors' appointments and treatments. But I witnessed amazing strength and courage. I'll never understand how Dad and Fran maintained such a positive attitude. Nearly every time I saw Fran, she asked, "How's Dad?" Sometimes my answer would be short. "Hanging in there." And at other times it would be rather lengthy. Dad was a very complicated case!

Now Fran and Dad knew each other, but not really well. This past winter, on the night of the Soo vs Petoskey boys' basketball game, Dad was shuffling out of the gym as Fran was sitting at the doorway in her wheelchair, sporting her pins that read "Please don't kiss me during flu season." Dad had become such a lover in his later years, and upon seeing Fran, he bent over and laid a big kiss on her. The next day, I apologized to her for Dad's lack of judgement. Fran's only response was, "I loved it!"

Dad's status deteriorated quickly mid-June, and on June 13, 2018, he went home from the hospital with hospice care. That very same day, Fran moved to Hiland Cottage. I visited briefly with Fran the next day on my way up to the UP. Of course, she asked, "How's Dad?" I replied, "Not well." We worked a deal. If she was to move on first, she would take Dad with her, and I would ask Dad to do the same. I spent the following weekend at Dad's bedside, praying for peace and comfort, not only for him, but for Fran, too. I made a quick trip to Petoskey on Monday, during which time I visited with Fran. Again, she asked about Dad. I reminded her of our deal; would she stop and grab Dad on her way? She smiled with as much of a smile as she could muster and shook her head "Yes." Dad passed away in the early morning of Wednesday, June 20, 2018. Fran passed away six hours later. Shortly after Dad passed, I witnessed two shooting stars. Coincidence? Maybe. But I choose to find comfort in the thought that Fran and Dad are walking and talking and maybe smooching a little and are in a much better place. I miss them both dearly, but I am so thankful for the lessons that I have learned from them both, to be selfless and strong, caring and courageous, kind and compassionate.

—Julie I.

How it all Began, How I Met Fran, the Sister of My Heart...

My husband Jeff and I met MaryFran and Andy Kolp in Lamaze classes while pregnant with our boys in 1999. Fran and I chatted about our impending births while the men were discussing the very important subject of bird hunting. From that moment on we were fast friends. Little did we know that was the start of a deep and long-lasting sisterhood.

Our sons, Hunter and Danny, were born one day apart. I had Hunter on June 13 at 5:00 p.m. Fran came in to visit at around 9 a.m., had an OB checkup, and came back to tell me they were going to induce her within the hour! Danny was born that day, June 14!

While I was pregnant with Kira, Fran asked me what I wanted for Christmas, and I told her to get pregnant again. Fran, being the good friend that she is, got me what I asked for! Kira and Megan, our daughters, are four months apart (Kira 4/25/01, Meg 8/30/01).

Fran and I raised our babies together like cousins. The Kolp kids call Jeff and me Uncle Jeff and Aunt Mel, and to my kids they are Uncle Andy and Aunt Fran. Since the kids were born, we probably saw each other or spoke on the phone every day for thirteen years. When the kids were babies, Fran and I took them everywhere together. Throughout the years our families celebrated holidays, birthdays, and took many family vacations together. In raising our kids together, we were truly sisters, sharing joys, concerns, and tough times. Just like sisters we were always there for each other, encouraging, laughing, fighting, crying, and constant. Fran and I played and worked out together, trying to get our bodies back in fighting shape. We started with spinning at Bentleys and moved on to road bike rides and sprint triathlons.

When it was time for school for the kids, Fran convinced

me to send the kids to St. Francis Xavier School despite us not being Catholic. What a great experience we had becoming part of the SFX family! During our time at SFX, I would describe my relationship with Fran as partners in crime. We taught extracurricular science together, volunteered for auctions and school functions, and even coached soccer together for a season for parks and recreation. When I say we volunteered (all of you know Franny), she signed "us" up; she was the big-picture lead and I was the follow through/detail person. Whatever it was we did together always turn out well, with a little chaos but loads of fun for all of us involved!

How Fran's ALS inspired us...

When Fran was diagnosed with ALS, Jeff and I had been in the middle of trying to decide if we would follow our dream of moving out West. Leave everything we knew? Move all the way across the country? Leave all our friends and our kids' friends and family? When we were hit with the reality of how life can change in an instant, our decision was made. This was the only time that would be right for our kids' lives to have an adventure like this. The time was now or never.

The guilt of leaving when your "sister" has been given this challenge is immense, let me tell you! But of course, like a true sister of the heart, Fran was the first to tell me to do it. "Go, follow your dream, and don't look back. We have our phones and planes." The experience out West has changed our whole family for the better and has brought us all closer together, I believe. Summers and vacations together are made even more special because our time with the Kolps meant more quality time versus quantity. We don't take our friendship for granted; we celebrate it.

More importantly, how Fran inspires me...

Fran, Franny, Aunt Fran has always been an inspiration to me in so many ways...

"Mel, just go with it." "We'll figure it out when we get there." "Plan ahead? What's that?" I was always worrying, and she was always "just winging it." She did help me learn not to sweat the small stuff so much.

"Let kids be kids." Letting the kids play in the mud in Porter Creek, letting the kids eat themselves silly, and most contentious— letting every kid at the birthday party stick their spoon anywhere they wanted into the birthday cake all at the same time! I would freak out at Fran's lax way of letting the kids do their thing, and Fran would crack up at how crazy I made myself trying to keep it all orderly. I think in the end we balanced each other out. My kids think, Thank goodness for Aunt Fran, the good cop.

"Everybody's got something going on." Sometimes when I was being critical or upset about another individual or a situation, Fran was always the first person to give them the benefit of the doubt or encourage forgiveness in saying, "You never know what else they have going on in their lives."

"Mel and I will do it!" Always the energizer bunny, Fran was up for anything, anywhere, anytime. Always willing to help a cause or person, Fran was the first to volunteer to get involved. Probably the biggest lesson, inspiration, gift Fran has given to me was her "you get what you give." Well, Fran, I feel so very blessed to have gotten you.

Thank you for everything, my beautiful friend, inspiration, and sister of my heart.

I love you,
Mel

Dear Fran,

I will never forget the day you informed me of the diagnosis that we all wanted to refuse. I will never forget your resolve to help others, help yourself, dig deep into your spiritual core, and become the strongest human being as your physical body weakened. But most of all, I will never forget the most amazing hours we spent together as I worked on you, trying to offer some bit of relief. All the conversations, laughter, tears (oh, the tears) regarding our families and most of all children are a gift I will treasure throughout my lifetime. The "sisterhood" of our community and beyond was brought together because of you. Fran, I promise to always share a memory of you every time I see Danny and Megan. And, I promise to never forget all that we shared, and how you helped me as I was trying to help you. YOU are and angel, Fran!

I Love You,
Shelley

MaryFran,
Your eyes shining bright
Your smiling face
Your arms opened wide
Your warm embrace

You make hearts feel alive
Loved and special
True gift from God
You Fran, are his Vessel

You touch many hearts
And spread God's cheer
You live well
Holding others dear

Spirited and free
Joy and energy abounds
That's our Frannie
With thought lots of people around!

You're a special friend, Fran
Soul sisters at heart
We are always close
Even when we're apart

From Birmingham to Toledo
Petoskey to GR
Sometimes close, sometimes far
But always connected, no matter where we are

We've dreamed dreams
We've shared goals and plans

We got engaged and married
Yes, we found our man!

Randy and Andy (or as I say, raggedy Andy!)
Teammates, classmates, roommates and more
Hunting buddies, basketball fans
Need I say more?

Yes, actually!

It's their roaring laughter and humor
Connection to the core
That warms our hearts
It's them together, we adore!

Through babies and bottles
Activities and sports
We did it all
With each other's support

Your words of wisdom
And encouraging advice
Has helped many through
Life's gripping vice

You are an entrepreneur
And athletic machine
Frannie the Organic
And inspiration Queen!

ALS has never beat you, Fran
You have fought more than well

The lessons I have learned through you
Have encouraged me to excel

I have learned that life is surely a gift
I only get one chance
So, I thought, what will I do
To make the most of my dance?

I will love on others
I will hug them tight
Make them feel special
With all my might

I will be understanding and grateful
Nonjudgmental and kind
For this is the way you work, Fran
Conscientious and refined

I will care well for myself
Eat well and work out
Go on adventures
And be proud of my route

I will live out my passion
To help change the world
Speak heart to heart
And give out life pearls
I will be courageous and fight
Through the good and the bad
Have faith God is with Me
No matter what is ahead

You are an angel God's
Send to share in His message
To live with passion and love
And to rise above the wreckage

You will always be close, Fran
No matter where you are
It goes without saying
You are a shining star!

—Paula

Dear Mrs. Kolp,

You are an inspiration. You are the strongest person I know. It amazes me how strong and kind you are despite the situation that you've been dealt. I know we haven't known each other for long, but I am so happy to have been in a little part of your life. You inspire me to live life to the fullest and recognize the blessings that I have been given. I wear your bracelet every day not just to support you on this journey, but to also serve as a reminder to not take the simplest things for granted. It was a great honor to have you be my NHS sponsor and I just want to thank you again. You have given me a different outlook on life and I want to thank you for that, as well. I love you.

Sincerely,
David P.

To MaryFran:

The other day my daughter was trying to teach her one-and-a-half-year-old daughter how to talk. My daughter said, "Say, 'Apple.'" And my granddaughter said, "Apple." Then my daughter said, "Say, 'Banana.'" And my granddaughter said, "Nana." Next my daughter said, "Say, 'Blueberry.'" And my granddaughter said, "Meow." This made me think of you.

I'm sure you're wondering why this made me think of you. Isn't it obvious? Just kidding. I'll explain. Sometimes in life our Heavenly Father/Teacher gives us a one-on-one lesson with His undivided attention. And sometimes a lesson is as simple as "Say, 'Apple.'" It's simple and easy to understand and we don't get it, no problem. Sometimes God's lesson is more like," Say, 'Banana.'" We kind of get it. We try our best, but we don't quite nail it. Thankfully, our Father/Teacher is patient with us.

Then there are times when our Father/Teacher says, "Say, 'Blueberry.'" At this point, some people begin to doubt the value of the lesson and even doubt the teacher himself. They decide they don't want this challenge. They don't want to learn this lesson. They don't trust the teacher. They say, "Meow." They back away from their lesson and their teacher. And sadly, they lose faith, never learning the depth and the width and the breadth of the love the teacher was hoping to impart with this particular lesson.

Every life is full of apples and bananas from time to time. Remember what we are taught. We remember who our teacher is, and we go on through life hopefully learning our lessons and sharing the wisdom we gain. You, MaryFran, have been here and the mother of all blueberries. Blueberries so big, so complex, so incredibly unfair, nobody can blame you if you decide to throw your paws up in the air and say, "Meow." Maybe even scratch up some furniture and pee on the couch a little, and I'm sure you have your moments of despair and anguish over all of this. And I'm sure there have been plenty times when you have struggled to understand how a loving Father/Teacher could possibly allow you such a challenge. We all have.

But, MaryFran, I have to tell you it is because your faith has not been broken that the story about my granddaughter made me think of you. It is because your faith has rooted itself even deeper in God's love for you, and His promise of everlasting life for you with Him and His kingdom that YOU have become OUR teacher. You are facing a challenge that would shake anyone's faith to the core. But your faith has grown branches. Branches that have reached out and touched everyone around you and throughout our whole community. Through all the things that make you "you," and most of all through your incredible faith in God the Father, Jesus Christ His Son, and the Holy Spirit, you, my friend, have taught us to ROAR!

Thank you!

—Jeanne Y.

My Michigan Hero

Have you ever had that one person who completely changed your life forever? I know a lot of people write about their moms, but I truly feel that she is the most important person in my life. Most kids do not face the things we do. My mom was diagnosed with a disease called ALS on her birthday, July 3, 2014. I have not thought about the fact it had on me until now. When I first heard about her diagnosis, I was a wreck for weeks. I would think, what will it be like to not have a mom? What will it be like to just have a dad? Why is it me? *Even just thinking that, I know there is no cure for what breaks my heart. She has such a spirit and an amazing sense of humor. You would not even notice that she has the disease because she pretends it does not exist.*

She is still there for me wherever, even though she is so busy with all of her treatments that help her work on trying to heal. It's like I'm a magnet and I pull her wherever I go, because she is always at my side. I know when she is there because I always get this warm feeling every day, like a lot of people do when they are with someone they love.

She will be at every one of my games, cheering me on and keeping me pumped up, but one day I feel like I will look over at the stands and see that she is not there. I had a dream like that and I walk downstairs and told my mom it was just a nightmare, and just held her in my arms, just saying to myself in my head that it will be okay. I couldn't stand not hugging her at that time. When I woke up from that dream, I felt like I lost everything.

I could have never been so close with anyone in my life. We act like sisters. She is the most honest and understanding person I know. I cannot believe life without her. She knows how to get the party started and keep it going. To be honest, my mom is the craziest and weirdest person I know. I feel like my friends love her more sometimes, though, because they all call her Mama

Kolp, Auntie Fran, and the best of all, Mom. Sometimes I feel like my friends just like me because of her.

When I grow up, I want to be a role model just like my mom. I cannot think of one person who does not love her. It is unbeliev-able. She is a hero to everyone. I think every day, I want to be just like her, not because I am forced to, because I want to.

—Megan K.

I met MaryFran Kolp in the summer before the 2013–2014 school year. It happened at an auction meeting in the parish office. I was immediately smitten and struck by MaryFran's uncanny skills and abilities. I knew right away that she was a phenom! I knew she could bring people together! The auction was at a crisis point at this time, and Father Danny had painted a grim picture of what we had for the auction, which is the critical fund-raiser for our school. MaryFran Kolp to the rescue! MaryFran took over and things immediately fell into place. She was energetic and provided the necessary leadership for all of us to climb on board. It was apparent to everyone that MaryFran had a magic, a special talent that the rest of us did not possess. We knew under her leadership that we could fix all the problems that we had with our auction. MaryFran made it happen. She practically lived at the school and she change the paradigm. One person, confident and willing to do whatever she could for the benefit of Saint Francis Xavier School, turned a struggling and potentially failing auction into a success. MaryFran Kolp has that kind of power and ability. She is a great leader, who led us by example, love, and an unceasing commitment. It's safe to say that MaryFran Kolp used all her skills, talents, and abilities to glorify God. She made a difference to our school!

—Jim K.

Mary Fran and I first bonded over the correct pronunciation of the word "data", which, as Fran would often point out (to me at least) was almost always pronounced incorrectly, a fact with which I completely agreed. So, Mary Fran, I will forever be your keeper of the proper pronunciation of "data".

Deb G.

Where do I begin to talk about someone you love so dearly that words are not enough to express your feelings? MaryFran is one such special person. A loving and devoted mother and wife, a born leader, and a good friend and confidante.

I first met Fran years ago when our kids studied at SFX. I got to know her better when she chaired the SFX auction not once but twice! I thought she was crazy, but she did it so naturally. She'll say she had a lot of good help. Well, as a great leader, she has a way of making you do your work and just be happy doing it! And she is smart as heck! Needless to say, those were the most successful SFX auctions we've ever had!

Fran and I were also with the Northern MI Alliance, a group of physicians' wives that participate in worthy causes.

Fran and I had a great time together when Danny joined USTA and played high school varsity tennis with my son Nico. We traveled, we laughed, we cheered. Fun and awesome time not just for our boys, but for us, too!

Fran has a deep love and faith in God. This unwavering faith has given her strength in mind, body, and spirit. It takes a lot of courage and strength in all aspects to deal with ALS, and she is doing a remarkable job. Such an inspiration. Starting her IV for IV infusions for several months was probably the hardest thing I have ever done. I hate needles myself (funny for an IVT nurse), but Fran just took it in stride. So brave. I think she was the one comforting me through this whole process, but it was a relief for both of us when it was over. Instead of dreading to see her, I now look forward to my every visit. Such special moments.

But what endeared me most to Fran is her personality. She sees the good in every person. She literally loves everyone. I have not heard her say anything negative about anyone. I think this is a remarkable trait because I am so guilty at times of doing the opposite. Fran is truly a beautiful person, inside and out. And I feel so honored and blessed to have known and met her in this lifetime.

—*Vanessa*

Ode to MaryFran

I believe I met MaryFran in a life "BK" (before kids), but only briefly, and we saw each other intermittently through the years at various events. I do remember thinking, Dang, those little kids are so tall, *in reference to her son and daughter! However, our friendship developed more deeply as she asked me to coach girls' basketball at St. Francis with her. One never said no to MaryFran, not because she is bossy, but because you love her so much and want to be around her all the time! Megan was in sixth grade at the time and playing on the seventh-grade team. We had so much fun and hopefully taught the girls along the way. The "short bus" rides were always fun, and lots of singing from the girls made the long trip to Rogers City less boring. I sometimes had to keep MaryFran composed so she wouldn't get a technical! However, I learned so much from her. She had an amazing relationship with all the girls and they were so blessed to have her as their coach. I learned things from her, as well, such as, "She's having a tea party under there!" In reference to how open a player was under the basket and nobody was passing her the ball. I still use it to this day! I now have the pleasure of coaching her daughter again, this time in high school on the varsity team. Megan is a talented, hardworking young woman and I know this is due to her mother's influence on her. I am so blessed to know and be friends with MaryFran and her wonderful family that she has nurtured, her immediate family as well as the community family that we have all become in being able to care for her and her family. The world will be quite dimmer when the light of her being is gone from this life.*

—Gina W.

How do I describe MaryFran Peterlin-Kolp and our friendship? I was introduced to MaryFran by Melody Collins. MaryFran and Melody had birthing classes together for the boys. Melody told me she and Jeff had met this really fun couple and that we should get to know them, too. However, it wasn't until MaryFran had her second child Megan, the same year that I had my daughter Genevieve, when we started hanging out more often.

MaryFran invited us to her music and movement class. What a hoot! MaryFran is a natural teacher. Around the same time, Melody told me that MaryFran was working on her doctorate and wanted to hire me to edit her thesis. I was working as a graduate advisor at the time but wouldn't let MaryFran hire me because I told her I would rather be friends. She told me she needed an editor more than a friend, and we actually managed to do both! I learned more about homocysteine levels than any non-medical person should, but I also learned how much MaryFran cares about others, especially children. Her study actually uncovered cardiovascular disease risks in several children. After that, I often address her as Dr. Kolp.

The first time she invited our family over for dinner, we had her famous Hawaiian chicken dish and my children were in heaven. Cats named after exotic Greek islands, dogs, pet mice, wild snowmobile rides, and romps through the woods looking for leeks. MaryFran refers to us as the city folk while they were the country folk.

MaryFran always enjoys getting moms together. It started with the music and movement class but quickly included duck races down Porter Creek or fireworks and barbecues at the lake. MaryFran and I had a fun mom-and-daughter weekend in Chicago for an American girl doll experience.

If there was a product that was healthy or improved a person's life, MaryFran got behind it. Who hasn't been to one of Fran's home parties? And every time there was a fund-raiser,

MaryFran's home business was the largest supporter. Several of my t-shirts have Drs. Kolp on the back.

MaryFran is also one of the founding members of the mom's organic cooking club. "Let's be healthy together and make family life easier" was her reasoning. Extra meals were always given to families with new babies or struggling through one of life's hard times. Little did she know the cooking club would be making meals for her family several years later.

Through volunteer experiences at Saint Francis Xavier, I witnessed MaryFran's leadership and dedication to service. Whether it was auction chair, PTO president, or class helper, MaryFran was always present. During our daughters' middle school years, it was fun to watch MaryFran's competitiveness and fiery nature reveal itself as a basketball coach.

MaryFran's birthday is July 3. It's usually difficult to celebrate because you can't live Up North without constantly hosting friends and family in the summer. However, we try to squeeze in some birthday cake during our annual Fourth of July Parade party. If we want to celebrate her birthday in the summer, she is a great sport about including all the summer birthdays. Because of this, I have been lucky to spend time with her wonderful extended family, too.

MaryFran doesn't like the spotlight on herself. She is definitely more comfortable on the giving end versus the receiving end. ALS stinks. I know she accepted the idea of Fran's Frantabulous Friends only because of Andy, Danny, and Meg. MaryFran is a beautiful friend who has allowed us all the opportunity to give back to her a small fraction of the love she shares with others.

—Maggie K.

MaryFran, when you came into my life, I immediately loved you as if I'd known you forever! But little did I know the impact you would have on my life. I will always remember your stories from high school, on long car rides home from tournaments, your open invitation to come and talk, and snow days spent watching Hallmark Christmas movies. Most of all, I will never forget the endless love and acceptance you showed me, and I can never thank you enough for that. You were taken from us too soon, but I know that you are somewhere better now. I will miss you always.

Love,
Kir Bear

One of my most memorable moment of you was when you came to my house to talk to my daughter Annie. She was going through a self-imagined phase and eating was becoming a problem. You sat in my kitchen and first told her how beautiful she was. She hears that from me all the time but hearing that from someone so confident and inspiring made all the difference in the world. After that, you just talked to her, and I mean really talked to her. She listened and so did you. Sometimes we hear people talk, but it takes a special person to really listen. That person was you. Words aren't enough to express my gratitude for what you did for my Annie.

When you ask me how your cross has affected me in a positive way...you have showed me humility. I hate when people say, "God only gives us what we can handle." I tell God that I am not as strong as His son is, but then there's you. You showed me that no matter how heavy my cross may be, God is there, with his angels, to help me carry it. Here's a prayer that my students and I say every day.

May the pure white light of God's perfect love surround you. And each step that you take, be guided down golden, protected pathways.

God's graces to you,
Kathy M.

Things I Learned from MaryFran Kolp
By Ashlee N.

- Kids need to fall to learn how to pick themselves up.
  - There was a time Danny made a comment he immediately regretted. He came to me after school to apologize. You later came to talk to me about the conversation the two of you had about it. I remember thinking that this was the way to raise a kid. He felt remorse, he wanted to talk to you about it, and he did what he could to make it right. You didn't make excuses for him, and you guided him through so that he learned from the experience. I will never forget that.

- Parents need to be parents.
  - There was a time when we were talking with another parent about whether or not her child would be going to the public middle school. She made the comment that it was about what her child wanted. You were not shy about how you felt about that. Children are not capable of making decisions regarding the rest of their lives; that's why they have parents. I not only respected your perspective, but I loved that you were not afraid to speak up.

- Sometimes you need to be loud to be heard.
  - My first-year coaching with you was the first year I was the "head" of the volleyball program. I had relied on Kim my first two years to know what to do, and then when it was on me, I was a little stuck. You showed me how to take charge.

- Try to make sense of God's plan.
  - Megan's eighth-grade year, right after you had been diagnosed, we were at Camp Daggett. It was one of the

first times I was able to talk with you. Your attitude was
unreal. You told me that you felt God gave you this so
someone else wouldn't have to go through it. Any time I
get frustrated or feel wronged in some way, I honestly think
of you. If you can look for understanding from God, then
so can I. What is He trying to teach me with the burdens he
places on me? How can I use them positively? Although
I've heard this type of advice my whole life, you are who I
saw personify it.

How do you honor your Mentor, your Hero, your First Friend, your Best Friend, your Sister...my sister MaryFran? How do you thank someone for having such an amazing impact on your life?

MaryFran was such a huge personality that she deserved to have multiple names: MaryFrances, MaryFran, Mary, Franny, Fran, Petie, Pete, and even Daddy Long Legs from her track star days. She was a celebrity in high school and carried so much clout that her nickname Pete (short for Peterlin) transcended to the rest of our family. Dad became Mr. Pete, mom was Mrs. Pete, and I became Re-Pete. Fran, of course, had sweatshirts made, because that's what she did, always going above and beyond. I called her Fran since I was young because I did not think she looked like a Mary, and MaryFran was a mouthful to say. Among all her names I feel honored to be the only person in the world who has the privilege of calling her my Big Sister. She was my very first friend and my best friend. She was always quick to tell me, "I loved you first," as we were friendly competitors at everything. Strangers would often ask mom if we were twins, and mom would say, "Yes, except they are three years apart."

We had a Norman Rockwell childhood—at least we thought so, eating dinner every night at 5 p.m., family of four, and a dog. As we grew older we started to think, Norman's dad probably didn't wear Birkenstocks with black socks (before it was cool), our mom and dad never let us watch cartoons, and Mrs. Rockwell probably did not serve a Paleo Diet and eat organic food before anyone knew what it was. We thought it was normal to do push-ups and sit-ups during commercials if the television happened to be on, ride bikes barefoot all summer until the mosquitos ran us into the house, swing from a rope high up in a tree and jumping into a pond, and snowmobile all day until the police pulled us over and would tell us we can't ride around town. Dad, we only flipped the snowmobile and crashed into each other one time; yep, just once.

We fought very little, and when we did it was out of boredom. I recall two tenacious times: once we were putting away dishes and the next thing I recall was Fran chasing me around the front yard with a spatula and a frying pan, then she locked me out of the house, and she won that battle. Being the little sister, I had to be more creative. I was tired of losing, so out of desperation I bit my arm and blamed it on Fran. She caught "heck" for that... and later that plan backfired because when I tried it again in a few weeks. I had recently lost a tooth, and my parents noticed the missing tooth in the bite mark. Darn...it's hard being the younger sister.

One of Fran's greatest traits was her ability to share and include others. She taught me to share and I was happy to share my Big Sister. She was also the Big Sis to my best high school friends (Michele Bird, Katie McCrary, Julie Nadeau, Paige O'Leary, and Shannon Oliver); none of them had big sisters and Fran was happy to oblige, offering advice on sports, being a captain on a team, applying makeup, high school, college, and boys. She taught us how to compete, earn college scholarships, be gracious young lady leaders, and how to have a little fun and not get caught. What happens at siblings' weekend at GVSU stays at GVSU.

I know I was Fran's best friend as we've always known we can count on each other for anything—any...thing. Our family is so small that we had to depend on each other. I also know that someone amazing as Fran would have multiple best friends. Her heart was so huge; she has room for all of them. Many of you here were her favorite for different things. I'm sure she had her favorite coffee mate, problem solver, decorating pal, travel companion, shopping partner, fund-raiser friend, beach-bum playmate, exercise buddy, high school friend, college pal, St. Francis best friend, and many more, and each of you knows who you are. Fran wore her heart on her sleeve and you always knew where you stood with her and how she felt about you. Only Fran could get away with telling you "how it was," whether you liked it or not, and you would thank her for setting you straight.

Fran had an exquisite way of making every moment count! She would turn the ordinary into extraordinary, like stopping by the park for the kids to play and grabbing ice cream on the way to the grocery store, or packing gourmet cheese, wine, and a fruit plate for a random sunset. If there was a birthday, anniversary, wedding/baby shower, graduation, or any momentous event, Fran would throw you a party and make you feel like royalty. She celebrated life and love at every opportunity! Our dad said it best: "Fran was only on this Earth for fifty years, but she LIVED 150 years!"

Fran loved to travel; she was always up for an adventure. Me: "Hey, Fran, want to go white-water rafting in W. Virginia?" Fran: "Yep." Me: "Hey, Fran, want to go island hoping in Greece?" Fran: "Sure!" Me: "Hey, Fran, want to go on a girl's trip to Vegas for Halloween?" Fran: "I'm in!" She wore her chicken costume on that trip and almost got kicked out of the casino. That girl was the best!

We traveled to Europe multiple times, a dozen trips to Florida as children, Las Vegas, Arizona, New York, California, and everything in between. In 1996, we were traveling in Greece with Fran's sister-in-law Nancy Finley and our dear friend Stefanie George, and it was my birthday. Fran hunted down a group of fraternity guys going to a college party and they were dressed as traditional grandmas dressed in house coats. Fran had them serenade me with birthday songs and dances. Fran always celebrated others, and if she really loves you she would embarrass you, too!

Fran succeeded at the highest level with everything she touched—college hurdle records that still stand, earning her doctorate, fund-raising record amounts for causes like St.

Francis Xavier Catholic Church. Fran never claimed perfection but was on a continuous quest for improvement. However, her greatest work was raising a gorgeous family. She gave them her all. So many of those who knew her are better people for witnessing MaryFran love on Andy, Danny, and Megan. Fran and Andy were the epitome of unconditional love. What a beautiful gift to provide Danny and Megan. What an incredible family! Fran was masterful with "Living in the Moment." We all continue to learn from her. MaryFran's courage, bravery, and faith are something imprinted on many of our hearts and live on in all of us. Thank you, Dr. MaryFran Peterlin Kolp.

Love always and forever past heaven,
—Natalie R.

I moved to Petoskey in 2005, and for the first time since being a mom, I could be a "stay-at-home mom!" My youngest son needed a preschool, and St. Francis Xavier School came highly recommended. Once enrolled the rest was history!

How I met MaryFran... Well, probably pretty much the same way anyone met MaryFran! "Good morning" or "Hi." "Welcome to Saint Francis. What's your name?" "There is a group of ladies that will be going for a walk after drop-off. You should join us." Or "There are a few ladies meeting at the Bistro, across the street, for breakfast. Please join me..." "I'm the PTO president. You should come to some of the meetings, and maybe you could run for PTO president next year. I can tell you would make a great leader" (or something like that). I was PTO president for the next two years. Ha-ha. Then there was the annual school fund-raiser that she headed for years, and yep, I was right there with her, willing to help in any way I could.

Fran organized a monthly "cooking club" at one of our local favorites, "Julienne Tomatoes." The club is still going strong today. Then there is the annual holiday, "white elephant" luncheon, and monthly birthday celebrations, held at Boyne Mountain's Solace spa... Life is good!

I may not have known MaryFran as long as some of the other angels in her life, but we grew close, quite fast. Her spirit and faith in God drew one to her. Her wisdom, knowledge, and calm demeanor were and still are exactly what one need when venting about some lame tragedy or female meltdown. We became friends who would walk, talk, bike, and quite often split a Greek omelet or some other meal. We even began working with a personal trainer, hoping to increase our strength and keep our adult figures looking more youthful! Helping each other push a little harder through push-ups, pull-ups, or planking, ugh.

MaryFran loved her personal business ventures. I was probably one of her favorite customers. There was Arbonne, Party

Lite Candles, Discovery Toys, Madison Hand Bags, and some I'm not even aware of.

In the middle of all her involvement with so many things outside her home, she still found time to make each and every holiday special in her home and for her family. I am in awe of all she was able to accomplish.

Some fondest memories include our trips to Mackinac Island for "Windsome Women," a Christian women's retreat. We went several years in a row, each with their own wonderful stories. (What happens on the Island, stays on the Island!) One year, we dropped the children off at school and headed for the retreat. Fran was driving, and on the way, we were pulled over for speeding! Our gabbing was quite distracting, apparently! Needless to say, the officer was kind enough to let us go with a warning. I mean, two sweet, kind, loving women, headed to a Christian retreat.

We could not be trusted…on one of our monthly trips to Gaylord, with a 30 percent off coupon to Kohl's, again our gabbing distracted the driver, me. Yep! We were pulled over for speeding. (By the way, no ticket.) We have grown wiser since then!

Anyway, as far as MaryFran goes, she has been the most amazing example of someone living a Christlike life! I have been encouraged by the way she has lived her life and continues to live her life, as she has suffered with such grace, strength, and determination. She has never once lost her faith in God and His will for us. We have no idea and never will have even the slightest understanding of our true potential as we live in this mortal state.

MaryFran is one of the most precious human beings I have ever had the privilege and honor to know, get to know, love, and learn to love from. My life has been blessed and enriched with

*her in it. Not much has been the same since that July 3 almost
four years ago. A journey that no one would wish upon another.*

*My continued, love, prayers, and support go out to MaryFran
and all her family.*

Xoxo,
Lynn

On the day I learned of Fran's death... Dan, Carole, Andy, Danny, Megan, Natalie, Josh, Sydney, and Ethan; Fran was many things to many people: a caring daughter, a loving wife, a devoted mother, a heroic sister, a doting aunt, and a friend to us all. My name is Mike Ewing and I stand before you as the representative friend of a family in grief, in a community in mourning, before a people in shock. Thank you for allowing me the opportunity to speak here today, a memory and honor that shall never fade. No human being could fail to be deeply moved by such a tribute as this. We've assembled from all walks of life and geography, not only in our desire to pay our respects to Mary Fran, but rather in our need to do so. She was the very essence of compassion, of duty, of style, of beauty. A true symbol of selfless humanity balanced wonderfully against a mischievous sense of humor with a laugh that bent you double. Fran's joy for life transmitted wherever she took her smile and boundless energy. She gave us strength in time of trouble, wisdom in time of uncertainty, and sharing in time of happiness. She will be by our side always. Love, loyalty, trust, and joy are not easy feelings to put into words, but she was all of these. She loved life completely and lived it intensely. Your attendance today is a testament to the type of person Fran was and the number of people she touched. While I do not know the dignity of Fran's birth, I do know the glory of her life. She died as she lived: unwavering, unquestioning, and uncomplaining. My estimate of Fran was made many, many years ago and has never changed. I regarded her then as I do now: as furnishing some of the most stainless examples of perseverance and determination. When I think of the dignified and dogged ways in which she managed her unsolicited health condition and fought tirelessly to rid herself of it, I am filled with a sense of admiration and humility that I cannot put into words and which will be with me always. She gave all that mortality could give and asked only in return that her loved ones and friends move forward in a positive and productive manner during her earthly absence. I for one intend to honor this request. Although I stand here to eulogize Fran, the truth is she needs no eulogy from me or any other man. She has written her own history and has written on the faces and in the hearts of Andy, Danny, Megan, and my dear friend Natalie. Through you all, Fran's spirit will live through eternity and any attempt by me to give a verbal legacy of her life is simply not possible. Today is our chance to say thank you for the ways you brightened our lives even though God granted you but little more than half a life. We will always feel cheated that you were taken from us, and yet we must learn to be grateful that you came along at all. Only now that you are gone do we truly appreciate what we are without, and we want you to know that life without you is very, very difficult. Unhappily, I possess neither that eloquence of diction, that poetry of imagination, nor that brilliance of metaphor to tell you all that Fran taught, but here is a glance at some of those teachings: 1. She taught us to be strong enough to know when we are weak and brave enough to know when we are afraid; 2. She taught us to be proud in honest failure, but humble and gentle in success; not to substitute words for action; not to seek the path of comfort but to face the stress of difficulty and challenge; to have a heart that is clean and a goal that is high and to possess a temperamental predominance of courage over timidity along with an appetite for adventure over love of ease; 3. Her endearing character created in our hearts a deep sense of wonder, the unfailing hope of what next, and the joy and inspiration for the deep springs of life. Now that she is gone, we are left to pick up the pieces as best we can, and in keeping with her wishes move forward in a positive direction. Her death leaves us with attempting to make sense of the senseless, to rationalize the irrational. This seems nearly an impossible task, so I can only conclude with full faith in my heart, and absent any reservation, that God called Fran home because his arsenal lacked a supervising Angel. I listen with thirsty ear for sounds of her laughter and her steadfast advice; in the evening of my memory I search for visions of her standing and cheering Danny and Megan to well-deserved sports victories. I would like to close by thanking God for the small mercies he has shown us at this dreadful time. For calling Fran when the pain was unbearable and the life quality nil; above all we give thanks for the life of a woman I am proud to call my friend, the unique, the complex, the extraordinary and irreplaceable Mary Fran, whose beauty both internal and external will never be extinguished from our hearts. Godspeed!

Delivered at Petoskey, June 25, 2018 (MCE)
—Mike

MaryFran, where do I start?

We met while pregnant with Danny and Sawyer, while our hubbies played basketball at Central School, twenty years ago.

My love affair for this person began right then and there. No matter who you are, MaryFran made you feel special and the only person in the room when she talked to you. You were special and what you had to say had importance. We had mommy tips and trips. We went on a few girl's campouts and man she could make me laugh. Never an unkind word.

We became fast friends, and golf partners. Kids played together and are still friends.

So on that day July 3rd when Sawyer was at Bay Harbor and asked Danny, "What's wrong man?"

He told him and Sawyer shared it with us. Sawyer came home sad and asked, "Mom, ALS is bad, right?" Who has ALS? God, I hoped he had got it wrong, like all of us. It's a bad dream, and so unfair.

Now given this diagnosis to a different person, it would have the same results. Give this diagnosis to MARYFRAN KOLP, look out people she will do all possible to find out how to fight this, while making everyone around her feel special and a gift from God. This TOWN and group of women found a way in "any way" they could to help. Again, all the while MaryFran made sure we were taking care of our families and ourselves.

Here's a funny story…

Doing treatments…

I took her downstate for treatments on one trip down,

I told her I need to stop and get me something to eat. I had Arby's and fed Fran her food Cheryl made for her each week. When I had finished my Arby's, I said, "Gosh, you must be hungry." She said, "Yeah, and you didn't offer me one French fry!"

I said, "Fran, I'm sorry. I didn't think you would cheat on the food plan."

She then replied, "I will cheat for a curly fry."
Oh we laughed. Love to hear the Kolp's laugh!
I remember when Princess Diana passed away, thinking to myself how sad but how lucky those boys were to have a mom like that, and what incredible boys she made and had left an imprint on their souls. Gone too soon! Like Diana, MaryFran left us too soon, but what amazing humans she created. Her spirit, kindness, and love are forever burned into my soul and everyone she touched.
I love you my dear friend

—Julianne K

My Fridays with Fran have been anything but boring. Every emotion—from laughter, tears, embarrassment, and anger—have come and gone during our time together, with unconditional love and respect the only constants.

Every week, I look forward to be a part of Fran's day and feel blessed beyond measure I've had this opportunity to learn about myself, my faith, and the true meaning of life. Fran has taught me invaluable lessons I will continue to carry with me always. She has modeled unwavering faith and a strong devotion to her family that have touched my heart. She is strong, determined, and wise. I am profoundly grateful for all her words of wisdom to me, particularly to me as a mom. There is no one in the world, or in my life, like MaryFran Kolp. Because of MaryFran, my faith now assures me God will continue to wrap His loving arms around Fran, her husband Andy, and their two beautiful children, Megan and Danny.

I met MaryFran through my dear friend and her sister-in-law, Terri Reynolds, about thirteen years ago. I learned quickly that Fran and I had two things in common—our birthdays (a day apart) and our husbands' extra-large shoe sizes. Fran's children, Danny and Megan, attended St. Francis Xavier, and it didn't take her long to recruit me to the PTO board. Somehow, my name ended up on the ballot even before my children attended the school. I blame Franny.

MaryFran has always a tendency to do whatever it takes to get families involved. I knew from the start that if I didn't want to participate in a project at St. Francis, I needed to avoid Fran at all costs. She has always looked at the spirit of service as a privilege and an honor, and it has always been her mission to cultivate this responsibility.

My Fridays with Fran started about a year after she was diagnosed with ALS. Our "Frantabulous Friends" all have different gifts and responsibilities, but keeping her clean, fresh, and smelling pretty was a promise I made to Fran right from the start. We both grew up with sisters, so showering together was never uncomfortable. What was a bit strange was when people stopped by to visit and "catch up" while we were in the shower together. It felt like a Seinfeld episode. Fran handled it with grace, and it gave us something to laugh about.

Poor Fran had to endure my weekly mishaps, such as dropping the shower head on top of her head, cutting strings that shouldn't have been cut, making her nose bleed by going too deep with the Kleenex, getting shampoo in her eyes, trying to use a razor blade to cut her cuticles, accidentally hitting her face with a hair dryer, and using a Q-tip wet with saliva to clean her nose. These are just a few of my mistakes. Fran just smiled and laughed at me. God certainly blessed her with patience.

The weekly showers were a regular for about two years, until recently. Weekly showers progressed to biweekly bed baths, prayer, and massage. I watched her decline physically, but by no means mentally. Every week her body became more fragile, but her faith has become stronger. I could tell what kind of day she was having by looking in her eyes. Watching someone you love suffer and lose more control every week is beyond difficult. I pray before I arrive at her home, and I pray when I leave. I ask God to use me as His hands and feet and heart to give me strength. It works.

Fran is an incredibly wise woman and has given me invaluable parenting advice and personal advice that I carry with me every day. She is beyond appreciative. She continuously thanks me with tears running down her face, telling me how grateful she is for making her feel "normal" and "not different," but the truth is, she's still the same Fran. She still makes the rules. She is in charge. She is still an amazing mom. She knows what she wanted and she is a wealth of information. Guaranteed, Fran knows more about me than I do. I remind her that if roles were reversed she would be heading up this fight for me. I also feel very strongly that the gifts she has given me outweigh anything I could ever give her. She has undoubtedly helped me put my life in perspective. I have learned to enjoy unloading the dishwasher and doing my laundry because I have hands that work. I don't sweat the small stuff anymore and my faith is a priority. It is what fuels me. God does have a plan, and it doesn't always go the way we want, but it's our job to put our worries in His hands.

Fran, you have taught me to HAVE FAITH, BE STRONG, BE POSITIVE, and GIVE BACK. Because of you, I now know for sure that our life here is temporary, so we'd better do this life right. Fran, you may be changing physically, but there's nothing about you on the inside—your beautiful strong spirit—that's changed. I love you, MaryFran Kolp. Thank you for being you.

Your friend always,
Jennifer

My name is Lisa P. I am one member of an amazing group of women that have had the opportunity to care for Fran and her family on her journey with ALS. Her journey is our journey, too. Along the way there has been great suffering and tears, questions, and even anger. However, there have also been abundant blessings, laughter, and sharing.

Part I: Meeting the "Famous" MaryFran

Although I lived in the area back in the 90s, I was thoroughly enjoying reacquainting myself with Petoskey as a "mom." It was 2013 and we have been in our new home for nearly seven months. Through my fifth-grade son David, I had made many new friends during Pop Warner football, travel basketball, and now lacrosse. One such friend was Lynn Rawson. Her son and David met during basketball season. Lynn is tall and very pretty, but more than anything else, warm and friendly.

As we got to know each other better cheering on our boys and all kinds of weather, Lynn spoke of her friend MaryFran. This woman described to me seemed to be superhuman. She worked out and went to church. She was a dynamic saleswoman, party planner, mom, volunteer, helper, and overall show runner! To top it all off, I was told she was tall, blonde, and beautiful. I imagined supermodel meets Martha Stewart. I thought she must be fearsome thing to behold!

And on a crisp and sunny Saturday in early spring, my husband Scott and I were excited for another riveting day of lacrosse, or as I saw it, an opportunity for more socializing! Lynn was near the entrance to the field with a friendly new face. As I approached, Lynn exclaimed, "Lisa, this is MaryFran, a friend I've been wanting you to meet!" Shit, I was not ready for this! My mind raced. What was I wearing? Did I curl my hair?

Do I have any makeup? Did I even brush my teeth? I'm sure I managed some kind of polite exchange while I scoped her out.

She was dynamic for sure, but also very warm and genuine. Almost instantaneously, I felt at ease. We only spoke briefly, but if she and Lynn went to their seats, I felt as though something special and extraordinary had just taken place.

Part II: Pink Pony Party of Four

It was the fall 2013. My husband Scott and I were planning to go to Mackinac Island for the weekend to celebrate a thirtieth birthday of a friend. The day before we were to leave, I ran into MaryFran in town. As we chitchatted, it was revealed that we'd both be on the island with our spouses on the same weekend! Even though I only met her once before, neither of us hesitated to try to arrange a time to meet up and get together.

On the island, our group enjoyed pub crawling and celebrating a milestone birthday. At dinner, I got a text from MaryFran. The plan was to meet later in the evening at the Pink Pony bar inside the Chippewa Hotel. At around 9 p.m., we made her way over and found MaryFran and her husband Andy (also known as Frandy), sitting on a wooden booth near the back of the room. We introduced the guys. I don't remember all that we talked about that night, but I know we had a blast! I remember laughing and Andy's distinctive laugh and worried we're going to get kicked out of the bar (those who know Andy get it!) Best of all, as we walked back to our hotel, Scott and I talked about how we cannot get over the feeling that we'd known Andy and Fran for 100 years.

Part III: Chicken Pot Pie and a Basketball Star

It was June 2014, and we were still reeling from the "Big Fall," as we called it. David had suffered a serious concussion after a twenty-five-foot fall from a rope swing. While laid up with stitches and a facial fracture, I tended to him and opened our door to many well-wishers and visitors. Having only been in Petoskey for two years, I was overwhelmed by how many people called or came by to see David.

*Somehow the word spread to MaryFran. Secured on our doorstep with a large bag from the Grand Traverse Pie Company, I was taken aback by her generosity, especially since we were still relative strangers who shared some laughs and a night out the previous fall. But there she was, offering us dinner, dessert, treats for David, and comfort. She inquired about David and asked if I needed anything. Now, normally I would politely say something like "thank you, we're all set" to someone I considered a new acquaintance. But at that very moment, I felt that **to know MaryFran is to love her, to be known by her, to be loved by her**. Her offer was genuine, and so for my needs, without hesitation, I told her that I needed someone to sit with David, so I could do some grocery shopping. Although she was attending to her own errands, she promised she'd soon return with her son Danny to stay with David. For David, this was better than all the gifts and visitors combined! For it was well known to all that Danny is the Michael Jordan of Petoskey and was on his way to basketball greatness in high school. David was already a huge fan, thrilled at the idea of Danny Kolp coming to our house!*

That third day after the accident was the turning point for David's healing from the "Big Fall," all through the kindness extended to us by MaryFran and Danny.

Part IV: I Have No Words

Life was slowly returning to normal after "the Big Fall." David had even been cleared to attend his Young Americans Camp sessions with some restrictions. The weather was warming up, the boat was in the water, and the promise of a fun summer was emerging. Then I got the call.

Lynn's voice sounded flat and drained on the phone as she relayed the devastating news. She spoke, and overwhelming sadness seemed to take the place of the oxygen in the room. I breathed it in and it saturated every part of me. Lynn continued to speak words my ears did not hear.

"Are you there?" she asked.

"I have no words," was my reply.

Later on, the day, my mind kept wandering back to MaryFran and her family. I thought about how devastated they must be, how scared they must feel. I thought of all the people who've known her for years, whose children grew alongside her own, and how they were trying to cope and share the news with their own kids. Lastly, I wondered how sad it was that I didn't get to know her more or have a chance to be close to her. If I could've only comforted myself then with what I have with her now, I just might have recognized all the blessings of ALS to come a little sooner than I did.

Part V: The Blessing of ALS

How could ALS lead to any form of a blessing? Humanity is an earthly realm and blessings are of the Kingdom of God. I had to separate the two in order, to answer this question.

When the news of Fran's diagnosis first broke out, the human part of me was angry. I questioned God. Why Fran, who gives so much to others? Why Fran, who has so much faith? Why Fran? The human part of me was sad. I was sad for her friends. I was sad for her family, husband, and kids. I was just sad. This was my human reaction.

Not long after Fran was diagnosed, I found myself on a trip downstate. Along the way, I saw three identical billboards—one in Elmira, one in Saginaw, and one in Detroit. They were Saint Faustina Sacred Heart of Jesus marked by these words, "Jesus, I trust in You." I felt as though they have been placed there just for me. On this trip, I had done a lot of "alone time" to think and reflect on all of this. My questions didn't all go away, but I took stock of these billboards and decided to trust Jesus. There are no answers to why Fran was stricken with ALS. No reason, but perhaps a purpose. Maybe she wasn't stricken with ALS but given ALS to bless the rest of us. This, in turn, changed my viewpoint. You could focus on the good that must come from this. This was my spiritual reaction.

Shortly after I returned home, a meeting of Fran's friends was held at Lynn's house on Walloon Lake. We all brought a dish to share and gathered to make a game plan for what lies ahead and how we can best support Fran, her family, and each other. At first there wasn't much to be done but pray. My involvement during the first two years was not as intensive as the last two years have been; however, she and her family were always close to my heart and I thought of them daily.

When I met MaryFran over five years ago, I could not imagine what our friendship would be like today. In my wildest dreams I could not have foreseen needing to feed, move, or wash her. Each new barrier we have crossed has been simultaneously uncomfortable, hysterical, and endearing. Not only did these situations bring us physically close, but spiritually and emotionally, as well. She is a forever friend and I am blessed to know her.

Today I live my life very differently than I did BK (before Kolps). Through my interactions with this amazing family in their journey, I became more grateful, kind, trusting, forgiving, and more aware of the presence of God in all things. I embrace each new opportunity with a jubilant "yes!" I say no to people and to things that do not lift me up or help me become a better version of myself. I do not miss weekly mass. I pray more. I seek to understand and look for the good in the worst of circumstances. I have been blessed with new friends and appreciate longtime friends with a renewed affection. I look to serve others before myself. Most of all, through MaryFran, I have witnessed absolute grace and strength in the face of the most, dire circumstances. She is like a living example of Jesus' suffering for our salvation. Her suffering is not in vain. It is a bridge to trust in God and accepting his blessings.

MaryFran,

I have written several versions of this letter, and even this one does not seem good enough. Your strength, character, and more wisdom have always been something I admired, long before ALS. When Kelly and Patrick were at St. Francis, we have such fond memories of how you were always smiling and treating them so well. Kelly said that no matter what, you always made a point of saying hi to her and looking her in the eyes. Patrick said that his SFX memory of you is you being in the lunchroom or playground and just having the warmest disposition, and everyone wanted to be around you. Kids are the best judge of character. Having an impact on children is something you can't fake; it's just who you are. I remember watching you coach basketball, and even if your team was losing, you were positive and had the ability to keep your players focused and motivated. Your presence at SFX was powerful, loving, and much needed. My family is blessed to have been at that school when you were a parent there.

I will never forget the day when we all gathered together at Lynn's cottage after we found out you were diagnosed with ALS. You came in all weak and feeble and the room got silent. You proceeded to say, "Just kidding. I'm not that bad!" Your sense of humor is fantastic, and you made us all feel so at ease. When my kids were going through sacrament prep, Sister Kathy would ask them to tell her about the times they saw God in their day. I see God through you; your faith is insurmountable. This disease doesn't make sense to me, but I know your faith in God is strong, which makes my faith strong.

I have not been as strong as a physical presence in your life and I wish I could have been, but please know that you have had my thoughts, prayers, and positive vibes for all these years. Thank you for always making me feel welcome around you and for being an inspiration of kindness, optimism, and faith.

You and Andy have raised two amazing children and their

near futures are really falling into place. We have a sarcastic saying at school: "The apple doesn't fall far from the tree." But in the Kolp family that's a blessing. Danny and Megan are hard-working, respectful, and kind kids—and that's because of who their parents are.

I love you and God bless you and your family.

Daily Catholic reflection from Matthew Kelly: What happens to you isn't nearly as important is how you respond to it.

Today's reflection 6/19/18:
"Just hold on one more moment. God is in control, even if it feels like he isn't he is in control, and he loves you. There are better things ahead."

—*Lisa L.*

Dear Fran,

I put off writing this letter because I have struggled with what to say. But here goes... I'm winging it at 5:30 in the morning, pre-coffee. The first time I saw you, you were standing with a group of mothers outside of the St. Francis school office. It was the first day of second grade for Danny and William. We had moved to Michigan in July; it had been a very rough two months at that point. I remember wondering if I would ever fit in, if the kids and I would ever make friends, and if it would ever feel like home here. Little did I know that the woman standing with that group of ladies with her hair in a ponytail, wiping little tears from her face as she laughed and talked (because she had just sent her daughter off to first grade), would become a force of nature and make me feel welcome. Within days, I would be asked all about myself and all about where I was from. I would be invited to boosters (let's face it, I went because I was desperate to get out of the house). During those first weeks, I heard your name over and over and over. "You've met MaryFran, right?" "MaryFran has talked to you, hasn't she?" MaryFran is the school welcoming committee. You led the other mothers in going out of their way in helping me through, what to that point, had been the hardest thing I've ever gone through. You hardly knew me, but within two months my kids, all three of them, were having sleepovers at your house. You are a force of nature that to this day draws people together.

During these days, I clearly recall a phone call by my brother. He was asking how we were all doing in Michigan. Were we meeting people? I told him that, yes, I was meeting the nicest bunch of people, that they are kind, welcoming, generous, and happy people. I told him this group of people were amazing, but I was baffled because, and I quote, "They are all friggin' Republicans." I never imagined being friends with people who are so far from my political thinking.

But here's the thing, MaryFran, you and I are on opposites in just about every way imaginable. You are athletic, a born leader, extroverted, social... a friggin' Republican. I am not any of these things. The thing with you is that you love in a huge way, and in my own way I do, too. I've never known anybody who is so able to make people feel loved. At the end of the day, that's all that matters. When you were first diagnosed with ALS, there was a flurry of activity of people sorting out how to help you. You have so many people around you who love you because you were simply so full of love. I have envied the talents of many of these ladies who seem to know what you needed, when you needed it. It took me time to be satisfied with my own way that I could make this whole thing easier, a little better...in the end it's you who was continuously teaching us all, not how to die, but how to live. Value every day, make time for things like vacations... We've seen so many states since July 2014. I've been wearing my "Be Brave" bracelet for four years; the meaning of it has changed for me. You've shown me that the best way to be brave is to turn everything over to God. Everything you have, you've given so graciously and in sickness, you have clearly shown so many of us how to live. Some people wear a lot of religious medals to remind them of their faith... For years to come I'll have my "Be Brave" bracelet, which makes me think of one of the loveliest, kindest, strongest friggin' Republicans I could ever hope to know.

I love you dearly, my friend, and I am ever grateful for you.

—Kathy

Theme from *The Courtship of Eddie's Father*, rewritten and performed
for MaryFran Kolp
by Marie L

People let me tell you 'bout our best friend
She's a warmhearted person
on her we can depend

People let me tell you 'bout our best friend
She's a right-brained fantabulous gal
through ups and downs she'll be your pal

People let me tell you about her—so much fun
Whether she's coaching man-to-man
or Whether she's talking one-to-one

She's our best friend
Yea, she's our best friend
LA-LA
ba-da-da-da-di-ya
ba-da-da-da-di-ya
ba-da-da-da-di-ya

She rocks an auction like 1-2-3, and we
teamed up for Springtime in old Pariee, Oui, oui!
Brushed up our game face and stayed carefree, C'est la vie

People let me tell you 'bout our best friend
She's a tall drink of water
with a taller son and daughter

People let me tell you 'bout her BFF
Andy's her one boy, cuddly toy
Their love produced their prides and joys

The day she saw him out there playing basketball
Her heart went boom-bah-boom-dah-boom,
With him she was enthralled

She said, "He is SO hot"
"We're gonna tie the knot"
LA-LA
ba-da-da-da-di-ya
ba-da-da-da-di-ya
ba-da-da-da-di-ya

She earned her Masters and PHD degree
She has great insight to share when I'm in need
Her faith inspires beyond belief, she's taught me...

Everyone she knows feels like her BEST friend
She'll often tell you, "You're the best."
And makes you better in the end.

People let me warn you, don't pronounce it "dadda"
It's one-of-those-little-things
that just drives-her-up-a-ladda

(Pause)

People it's no secret, Fran is one tough miss
Yea, from taking on the big boys down to fighting ALS

THE HIGHEST HURDLE

It's so sur-real
A crappy deal
LA-LA
ba-da-da-da-di-ya
ba-da-da-da-di-ya
LA-LA-LA-LA-LA

And every angel atop a Christmas tree
Now bares your smart-a&& smile, at least, for me
Forever grateful, I am, to call you my friend
My best friend

I first met MaryFran at St. Francis School in Petoskey, where we both did playground duty. Megan was a toddler and Danny had just started school. I came to know MaryFran as a woman with not only physical beauty, but also an inner grace and gusto for life that led her to chair multiple events at school while engaging in more than one entrepreneurial endeavor at one time. All this was accomplished while wearing the rewarding but challenging gift of the hat of mother.

Along with Andy, MaryFran continues to guide her children to recognize their gift of athletic prowess, refining it as it carries them to greater and greater successes. MaryFran inspires me to reach for multiple goals at once, with enthusiasm and encouragement for others along the way. The group of ladies that gathered around MaryFran at the beginning of her illness and continues to ride the undulating waves of laughter, sadness, prayer, and solidarity is a lifeboat that will never sink, but will inspire future generations of faith-filled sailors.

—Mary H.

By nature, I'm very care-taking.
There's something really beautiful about cooking for
someone and feeding them.
—Eric Balfour

This is a quote I found regarding feeding people. It summed me up beautifully because I do very much like caring for people, and in particular feeding them. Cooking and love of food found me after recognizing that my family art gene had been utterly absent, or at least badly mutated in me. I cannot draw a straight line or a normal-looking circle. Somewhere along the way I realized I can cook the apple, not draw it. Spatula replaces pencil and eureka!

I had known Fran for many years and shared many tears, laughter, and walks with her. She was a tremendous cheerleader of a friend, encouraging in a way that made one believe that they could actually do anything. It was my pleasure to be a part of her life and especially a part of her trial. She decided on a ketogenic diet—lots of fat, some protein, and a little carbohydrate—all organic. It is a very anti-inflammatory diet, and as it turns out, very yummy. First ingredient: butter! Let's face it, fat is delicious! I had a wonderful time week after week making her different foods, from Italian to Thai to Polish, all following the mandates of the diet and all high in nutrition with a lot of vegetables, all organic. As her disease progressed, we landed on a few very calorie-dense soups, shakes, and custards that were easy to swallow and sustaining. I can cook for anyone, but I fed Fran. I shopped for it, prepared it, sat with her and fed it to her, and it transformed me. When you hear about spiritual food, food for the soul, well, that kind of nourishment comes from serving others. I am improved by far in every way because she asked, and I answered.

Following are a few recipes that were critically beneficial when Fran had progressed. She no longer desired variety; her tastes were hypersensitive, and they were easy to swallow. One is Green Soup, a vegetable-loaded soup high in potassium and magnesium. It is not a pretty soup but don't let it fool you. I have a pot on now while I write this, and I eat it all the time. The others are her shake base and custard.

Green Soup

1 stick of butter
2 leeks, cleaned and chopped
4 large garlic cloves
2 large zucchinis, chopped
1 large bag of frozen spinach or kale
1 8-oz. container of sliced mushrooms
1 box of chicken broth or bone broth plus water
2 tsp of organic Better Than Bouillon Chicken Base
1 tablespoon of dried dill

Melt the butter in a large stock pot. Add all of the vegetables and sauté until they become a little brown. Add the broth plus enough water to just cover the chunks. Add the base and dill, and pepper if you like. Bring to a boil and then reduce and simmer for thirty minutes, until everything is soft. Cool and puree in blender. If you are eating dairy, add some heavy cream at this point. This soup freezes well.

Shake Base

In a blender, put:
1 can full-fat coconut milk
2 cans of milk of choice (cow, almond, coconut, cashew...)
2 scoops of high-quality vanilla protein powder
Store in a pitcher, and when needed, add any of the following:

frozen fruit, nub of banana, spinach, frozen cauliflower, unsweet-
ened cocoa powder, and almond extract...

Franacotta

Panna cotta is an Italian uncooked custard that uses gelatin to
thicken it. This can be made chocolate by adding cocoa powder
or chocolate protein powder. It really is a blank canvas—flavor
at will!

1 can full-fat coconut milk
1 can of milk of choice
1-2 scoops of vanilla protein powder
Stevia to taste to sweeten
1 tsp of vanilla extract
1 packet of gelatin

Put three tablespoons of water in a shallow bowl. Sprinkle
the gelatin on top and let it soften. In a soup pot, heat the milks
to a simmer. Whisk the gelatin and add it to the pot along with
the protein powder and sweetener. Whisk well and cook for five
more minutes. Remove from heat and whisk in vanilla. Pour into
ramekins (we used mason jam jars with lids) and chill until firm.
If you like it firmer, add a little more gelatin. While I did not
try it, you can freeze this. If you have a problem with it setting,
return it to the pan, add a little more softened gelatin, and heat
again, whisking.
Peace be with you and with Fran.

—Cheryl H.

I met Fran at St. Francis School in our hometown of Petoskey. She was always so welcoming and just so sweet. She was also so incredibly active in many fund-raisers for our parish, always giving back. I knew her—not very well—but I was aware of the struggles and weaknesses that she was having before she was even diagnosed. From the beginning MaryFran was going to fight the diagnosis no matter what and she sure fought an amazing battle. I promised her I would help her with whatever she needed. I had a nursing degree and worked in the ICU for a long time, but had never cared for an ALS patient. This was a journey for me, too.

Taking care of people is what I do best, doing God's work. There was a ton of us who decided that we are going to help Fran along this journey—be her warriors! When Fantabulous friends was started to help Fran, I was all in. It was such a great idea! Here is where the beginning of mine and Fran's friendship started.

My days with Fran went from helping her around the house, to helping her eat, to getting her medications together and counted them out for the next seven days, to ordering anything she wanted from Amazon, to talking about God, to showering her, toileting her, taking her to acupuncture, to giving her shots and starting her IV's, to finding the right medical equipment that could make her life easier. We talked about everything and anything.

I started with helping her in the shower because her left arm went first; it was hanging at the side of her body and her other was becoming weak, too. So, I started going into the shower with her. My friend Jen and I alternated days. I would undress and get her in the shower. I would wear my underwear and a sports bra. I would joke as I would wash her. We had certain code phrases that would give her a heads up on what I would wash next. I would shave her legs and wash your hair, towel her off, and get her dressed.

Things got harder as time went on. My friend Jen and I needed to shower her together. It was becoming unsafe to do it by ourselves. I never thought I'd be sharing a shower with another woman, let alone two other women, LOL.

As Fran's weakness grew worse she got more and more claustrophobic, and we would have to shower her with the door open. The showers turned into a race against the clock. Fran wanted to be done as quickly as possible; she would get very panicky. We were blessed with a shower chair that Jen had gotten from her father-in-law, and Jen and I had a good routine down. We would have the towels all set and ready, the chair ready for her to sit down after her shower. We would dry her, dress her, and do her hair and whatever facial treatment she needed. She absolutely loved having her ears cleaned. She always said the ALS made her hears itch something awful. During all this, we three would laugh, cry, crack jokes, and share intimate details of our lives.

Eventually, we had to give Fran a bed bath instead of the shower. She just didn't have the energy or muscle strength to stay sitting upright, and her breathing was easily labored with activity. We could still get her up to a bedside commode; I was pretty amazed at Fran's ability to still stand and walk with help. Her legs were weak and her balance off, but she could still do it, almost till the end.

Watching Frannie slowly lose so many functions and her ability to do anything for herself was heart breaking. Many, many times Jen and I would leave after our morning of Fran care and cry. Thru it all, she remained so faithful and never said, "Why me?" Every day I visited, I would enter her bedroom, hop into bed with her, and she and I would talk and pray. She always wanted to know what kind of things were going on in my life, my family. She was always telling me she prayed for me all the time.

She worried about me; that was her nature. She made sure, all the time, it was not all about her. Such an amazing lady!

I feel so blessed to have known Fran, to call her my friend, and to have spent time with her during her journey. Sadly, I didn't really get to say good-bye. My father was also ill and I went downstate to care for him and was gone when Fran passed. She slipped out of this life and into heaven four days after my dad did. I had a feeling when I last saw Fran that it was going to be the last. I think she did, too.

Since Fran has been gone, it's been weird going back to a schedule without her and her family. Every time I drive by her house, I feel pulled to turn in. I miss her, the kids, and coffee time with Andy, her amazing husband. God bless her and them. She was truly one of the wisest and giving persons I have ever met.

Mary Fran, you will be greatly missed but never forgotten.

Hugs to you, Kolp family! With the blessing of knowing MaryFran, I also got to know and love you all!

—Cheryl E.

ACKNOWLEDGEMENTS

I sincerely hope that you have fallen in love with MaryFran the way almost everyone she has come in contact with. I hope that this will help your journey in some small way if you or a loved one has received the diagnosis of ALS. Know that every day since her diagnosis, she has prayed that no one else would receive this disease, and that she felt she was given this diagnosis because maybe someone else could not have handled it. My own thoughts are that God chose her because He needed her to plan some parties up in heaven, and that He needed another person to help Him bring people together. That is the only way I am able to understand her diagnosis.

I leave you with this. Here comes the preachy part, so hold on! I promise it won't be too bad. Live your life as MaryFran did. Smile! Hug someone! Give a compliment! Tell someone you love them! Be kind! Life is short—make the most of it.

There are way too many people to thank for this book. The most important are my husband Fred, who is a saint for putting up with me; MaryFran's husband Andy, who is a special kind of person who loved her and worshipped her through the worst; my son Kevin and my daughter-in-law Sarah for their suggestions; my son John, who had to patiently wait for me for many days as I was helping MaryFran, and who always told me, "It's okay, Mom, you are helping MaryFran"; Danny and Megan, your mom loves you more than anything; and Deanna for always being there for me.

If we tried to list everyone we know, we would miss someone and that would break MaryFran's heart. So, if you brought a meal, a card, fed MaryFran, sat with her, rubbed her feet, bathed her, or basically helped the family in any way through her ALS journey or were a member of the Frantabulous Friends—she thanks you from the bottom of her heart and know that she loves you eternally. She calls all of you her angels and know that she is now our guardian angel.

—Kim